Helping Yourself with Foot Reflexology

Helping Yourself with Foot Reflexology

Mildred
Carter

Parker Publishing Company, Inc.
West Nyack, N. Y.

PRINTED IN THE UNITED STATES OF AMERICA

B & P (13-386680-7)

To my family
who, sorely neglected, stand
patiently by while I pursue
my study and writing.

Acknowledgments

My grateful thanks to my friend Martha Lanser for her valuable help in typing, and also to Emma Leah Handy for her typing.

I am also indebted to Barbara Batt for her invaluable help in drawing the charts for this manuscript, to my daughter Tammy Nelson for her patience in posing for photographs, and especially to Hilda Peterson for her help in getting this manuscript into shape.

Foreword

During my 48 years as a physiotherapist in my own treatment centers, as well as in some of the large sanitariums including Battle Creek of Dr. John Harvey Kellogg fame, I have had every opportunity to observe the amazing benefits of manual massage. As a means of rehabilitation where physical trauma is involved, it ranks high in the annals of medicine.

The techniques described in Mrs. Carter's book are not something entirely new but have been in use for many years. They do not replace, nor are they a substitute for, medical care under a physician. However, the use of reflex therapy, administered by the patient himself in most cases, by the simple manipulation of prescribed areas of the feet and hands, relieves tensions and similar psychosomatic conditions to an amazing extent.

The techniques described in Mrs. Carter's book have been developed by experts in the field of reflex massage, and we have no hesitation in recommending them to those suffering from the strains and stresses of modern living. For the relief of pain, we know of no other means short of opiates to achieve this objective.

CLARENCE R. MUNROE
Registered Technician, Physiotherapy

What This Book Can Do for You

The various organs, nerves, and glands in your body are connected with certain "reflex areas" on the bottoms of your feet, such as the soles, toes, and ankles. This book shows you how easily possible it is for you, through massaging these reflex areas in certain simple ways known as "reflexology," to activate natural and prompt relief from practically all your aches and pains. It is also possible through simple reflexology techniques, as demonstrated in this book, to help get rid of practically all types of poor health situations, and often help heal chronic cases that have not yielded completely through other methods of healing.

Moreover, reflexology can be used to keep yourself in good health; as a means of recognizing certain health problems before they may become serious for you; build resistance to attacks of disease; get more youthful energy; achieve protection from health-destroying mental and physical tensions.

Self-help reflexology techniques are described and programmed for specific health situations in simple steps, fully illustrated by diagrams and photographs as to how you can most effectively massage the reflexes in your feet. Each reflexology technique, as applied by you, has a direct effect upon the glands, nerves, and organs in your body. The indicated reflexology technique for simple manipulation of these reflex "buttons" on the bottoms of your feet can "signal" an attack or presence of a malfunction in a certain part of the body. The recommended reflex technique sends a surge of activity or stimulation where needed to help clear out congestion or certain other conditions and restores normal functioning. Helping yourself with reflexology involves no extra expense as there is no equipment nor anything special to buy.

Application of reflexology techniques may be made at your convenience at any time and practically any place. For example, if you wish to take a "reflexology break" for a fast pickup of energy, recharge of vitality, or to take care of a headache, etc., — you can do so at your office, in your automobile, while watching TV at home, even while visiting, and take only a few minutes to get beneficial results.

A glance at the index will indicate to you the wide range of situations for which reflexology has been used to get significant and concrete benefits and results as regards your good health. Case histories are set out that the author has encountered in her years of practice of the healing art of reflexology, and you will see what reflexology has been able to accomplish.

Reflexology is Nature's "push-button" secret for vibrant health, more dynamic living, abundant personal energy, better living without pain. You can get all these benefits, and even more, by keeping this book within easy reach for reference when confronted with a health situation.

Mildred Carter

Contents

Helping Yourself with
Foot Reflexology

CHAPTER 1

How Reflexology Works

Reflexology is a scientific technique of massage, that has a definite effect on the normal functioning of all parts of the body.

The late Dr. William F. Fitzgerald discovered the fact that pressure and stroking of certain reflexes would bring about the normal functioning of a specific location or organ in the body, no matter how remote it was from the reflex being pressed. He brought his discovery to the attention of the medical profession in 1913.

Eunice D. Ingham has blazed a path to this unique way to health through her many years of work and association with practicing physicians, on which the foundation theory of this work was set forth.

It was my good fortune to have studied under Eunice Ingham. I am grateful to her for enabling me to bring relief to so many suffering people and to have watched their joy in regaining health and vitality when all hope had been seemingly lost.

Now I give you this simple, unique, but scientific method of bringing health and vitality into your own life.

Healing Forces Released Through Reflexology

You will use the healing forces of Nature to revive glandular vitality. "The fountain of youth is within you." You can actually help yourself to beauty and health through the use of reflexology.

You can get almost immediate relief from many aches and pains by pressing a certain reflex button under the skin of your foot or hand, and massaging it a few moments in a certain way.

Most headaches may vanish almost immediately by manipulating the big toes, as they contain the reflexes to the head.

I have seen badly twisted hands and feet, caused from painful arthritis, straightened back to normal as a result of massaging the reflexes.

Reflexology can send Nature's healing forces to help a failing heart. It can stop the pain of hemorrhoids almost immediately, and cure a sore throat in a minimum of time.

Reflexology Usable by Anyone

This book will show you by way of pictures and charts, a simple method of how to massage these reflexes to bring relief of pains and diseases.

Not only will you learn how to distinguish and cope with many illnesses, and aches and pains, but also you will discover how to bring relief, and in many cases complete healings, by the simple technique of massaging the reflexes.

You will be able to slow the advance of old age and senility. By the correct use of reflex massage you can reactivate the body's natural process of rejuvenation and regeneration of cells, and bring new life to those who are already senile.

You will relax the nervous tension of your body and be able to sleep. You will be able to relieve others of pain and illness, through the blessed use of reflex massage.

You will learn the relationship of glands, and the influence they have on your health, your mentality, your life.

Reflexology will free you from sickness and suffering, and fear of pain, *when used correctly.*

This book will open the door to a different, scientific way to health, vitality, and the joy of living.

You will learn the power of thoughts concerning your health, beauty, and happiness. To be happy is to be healthy and beautiful.

Sadness, anger, and fear, create tension, which results in sickness and rapid aging. Reflexology relaxes tension. This book can guide anyone who can follow simple instructions to better health.

CHAPTER 2

Guide to Reflexology
Charts for the Body

Let us briefly study the charts of reflexology as they follow below for a moment, to get acquainted with the positions of the reflexes in the feet and their corresponding relation to the vital parts of the body. All diagrams in the feet represent *reflex areas*.

Explanation of Chart 1 (Page 4)

Look closely at Chart 1. Notice how the right foot corresponds to the right side of the body; the left foot corresponds to the left side of the body, when they are shown in a like proportion. If you get a clear picture of this in your mind, then it will be simpler for you to find the reflexes in your feet when you are learning to massage them.

It will become natural for you to know the position of each reflex and its corresponding part in the body, after you have practiced massaging the reflexes a few times.

Notice how the head corresponds with the big toe, and the position of the pituitary gland in the head. Now look at the reflex to the pituitary gland, in the center of the big toe. The pituitary gland in the head will be stimulated by massaging the corresponding position in the toe. Since the reflex to this gland is in the center of the head, you will massage the reflex in both the right and the left toe.

The neck and throat correspond with the base of the large toe

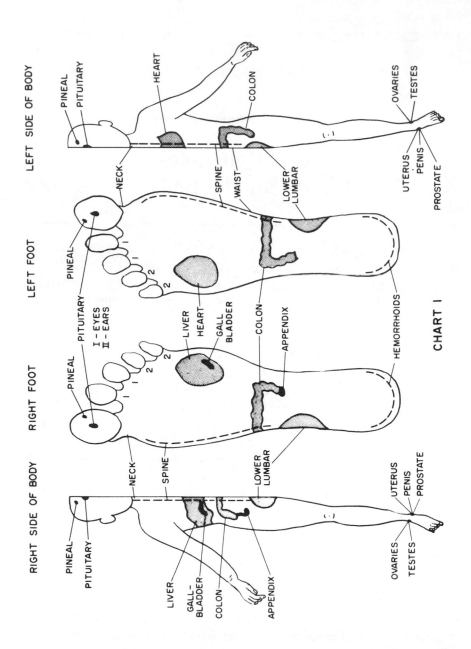

CHART I

where it is fastened onto the foot. The back of the neck and the back of the head will have reflexes on the top of the big toe.

As we progress down the body we will see how the spine corresponds with the bones along the inside of the foot, from the base of the big toe down to the heel bone. At the end of the spine in the body we likewise come to the end of the bony structure in the foot. If there is pain in the center of the back, you would massage the center of this bony structure in the foot (see the positions on the chart). If there is a centralized pain of the spine, you will not have any difficulty finding the right location of the reflex to it on the foot, as you will find it very tender as you press on it.

Let us now look at the toes. Notice that the eye and ear reflexes are just below the smaller toes. Since we have an eye and ear on each side of the head, there will be reflexes on each foot. The reflexes on the left foot go to the left eye and ear; the reflexes on the right foot go to the right eye and ear.

Notice how the liver is on the right side of the body and the reflexes to the liver are on the right foot, in a somewhat similar position. The heart is on the left side of the body; on the chart you see the reflex to the heart in a corresponding area on the left side of the foot.

We see the appendix on the right side of the body at the beginning of the colon, under the liver; the corresponding reflex to the appendix is on the right foot, below the liver reflex.

You should now be getting a general idea of how the position of the reflexes in the feet corresponds to the location of the organs and glands of the body.

Explanation of Chart 2 (Page 6)

Let us now take a look at Chart 2 for a fuller understanding of your body and the corresponding reflexes in your feet.

On this chart you will find the stomach and its reflexes, the colon, bladder, spleen, etc. Study it until you have the location of the organs somewhat fixed in your mind, in accordance with the reflex to each one.

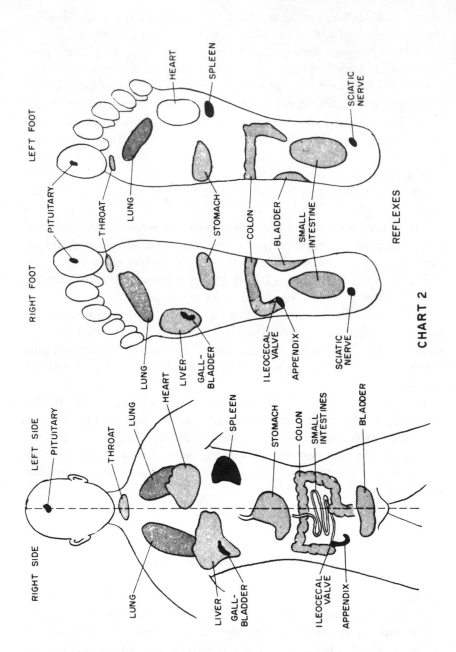

LEFT FOOT

HEART

SPLEEN

SCIATIC NERVE

PITUITARY

THROAT

LUNG

STOMACH

COLON

BLADDER

SMALL INTESTINE

REFLEXES

RIGHT FOOT

LUNG

HEART

LIVER

GALL-BLADDER

ILEOCECAL VALVE

APPENDIX

SCIATIC NERVE

CHART 2

LEFT SIDE

PITUITARY

THROAT

LUNG

SPLEEN

STOMACH

COLON

SMALL INTESTINES

BLADDER

RIGHT SIDE

LUNG

LIVER

GALL-BLADDER

ILEOCECAL VALVE

APPENDIX

Explanation of Chart 3 (Page 8)

Chart 3 shows the all-important endocrine glands which secrete the hormones into the body, and part of their various reflexes. You will be learning much about these in the ensuing chapters.

Explanation of Chart 4 (Page 9)

Chart 4 shows an area on the feet for reflexes that are centered more around the ankle. Notice that the gonads (sex glands) reflexes are not on the bottoms of the feet like the reflexes to most of the organs of the body. As these glands are most important to your health, this area should always be massaged a few moments whenever you massage your feet.

Summary of Charts

After studying these charts, you can understand how massaging the reflexes in your feet will stimulate the whole body. You will not be treating just one congested area; you will be sending an invigorating, life-giving flow of circulation to every part of the body. Following are illustrations for various positions you can take for massaging the foot reflexes (see pages 10, 11, and 12).

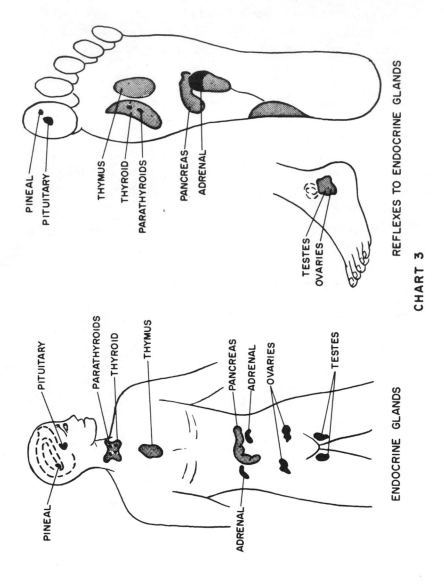

PINEAL
PITUITARY
THYMUS
THYROID
PARATHYROIDS
PANCREAS
ADRENAL

TESTES
OVARIES

REFLEXES TO ENDOCRINE GLANDS

CHART 3

PITUITARY
PARATHYROIDS
THYROID
THYMUS
PANCREAS
ADRENAL
OVARIES
TESTES
PINEAL
ADRENAL

ENDOCRINE GLANDS

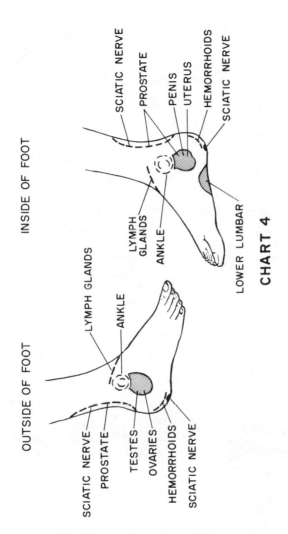

OUTSIDE OF FOOT

INSIDE OF FOOT

SCIATIC NERVE
PROSTATE
TESTES
OVARIES
HEMORRHOIDS
SCIATIC NERVE

LYMPH GLANDS
ANKLE

SCIATIC NERVE
PROSTATE
PENIS
UTERUS
HEMORRHOIDS
SCIATIC NERVE

LYMPH GLANDS
ANKLE

LOWER LUMBAR

CHART 4

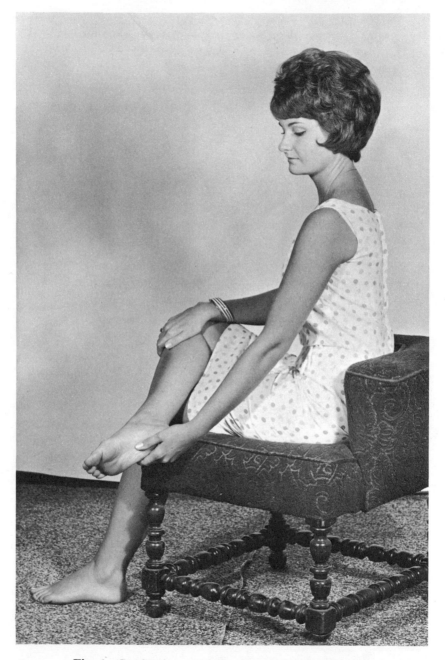

Fig. 1. Getting into position to massage the reflexes in the feet.

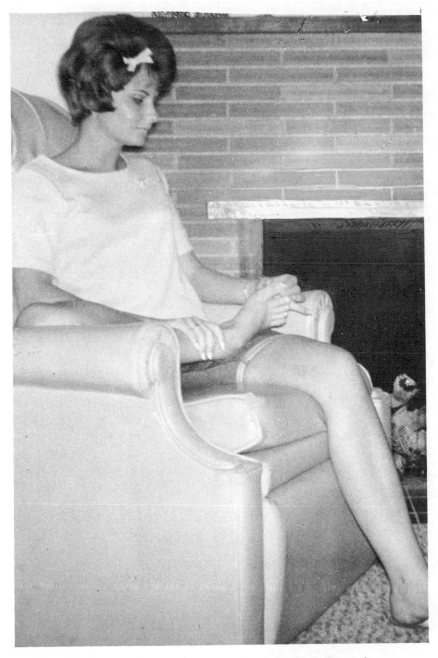

Fig. 2. A comfortable way to massage the reflexes in the feet.

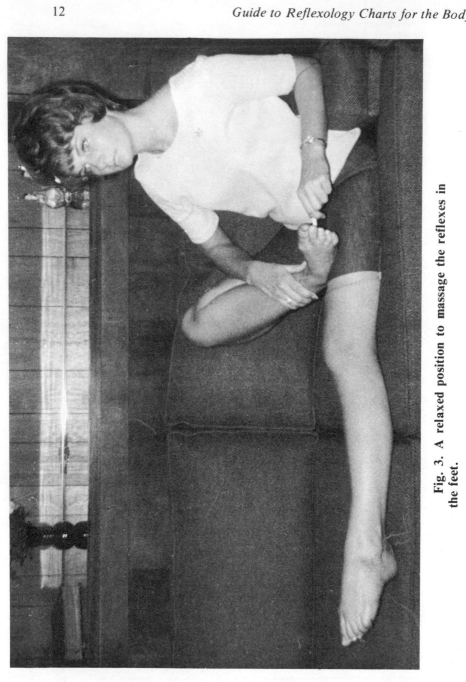

Fig. 3. A relaxed position to massage the reflexes in the feet.

CHAPTER 3

The Benefits of Reflex Massage

There is an ancient Arabian proverb which says, "He who has health, has hope; and he who has hope, has everything."

Probably no one would agree to this as readily and enthusiastically as the person who is ill, for usually one must know sickness before one is able to appreciate a sound body.

If retaining or regaining health were a single process, following along one definite line of endeavor or due to one specific habit, pursuing it would be a simple procedure. But in order to live abundantly, fully, with clear mind and vibrant body, so many factors are involved that every person should be constantly alert to avail himself of these means to enable him to get the most out of his years on earth.

God called His work good, and justly so, for not only did He create a marvelous body for man, but He placed the wherewithal upon the earth so man could remain healthy and happy.

Electrical Nature of Reflexes

One of the most miraculous means given man, and probably one of the least familiar to him, are the electrical reflexes in the bottoms of the feet and in the palms of the hands which correspond to every part of the human body!

These were placed there in the beginning when man was made to go naked, walking on his bare feet over rugged terrain.

13

Early man roved over plains, through forests, and stepped on sharp objects which pressed into his feet, reaching the tiny electrical reflexes, furnishing a natural massage. This natural form of massage broke and loosened any small crystals that might have formed there in the nerve structures or blood vessels, causing congestion, which would, in turn, slow the flow of blood to the part of the body corresponding to the reflex involved. The electrical shock stimulated the portion of the body for which that part of the foot was responsible, and the body as a whole was in rhythm with the universe.

Why Early Man Was Healthier

Early man was healthy because of this natural massage during his daily activities. When blood is slowed in any place by an obstruction, that place or organ becomes sluggish, just as a pond becomes stagnant when running water no longer flows through it.

Today we have footwear. We have sidewalks. We have smooth, soft, green lawns. Consequently, this natural stimulation of old *is no more*. But this does not mean that modern man must forego its benefits.

He is quite capable of managing this stimulation, either manually or by use of a hand "Reflex Massager" which comes complete with a book of diagrams and explicit directions.

There are so many personal experiences which I could recount, stories of numerous and interesting illnesses relieved by me through the use of massage that I find myself wanting to tell all of them at once. Massage is so simple and natural that it is safe to use on anyone from the youngest baby to the eldest person. And the benefits of massage? They are positive.

Author's Husband Struck with Heart Attack

As is so often the case, tragedy brought about my original interest in the matter of achieving good health. My husband was struck down with a heart attack when he was only 34. There had been no warning which we recognized at least, and the doctors at that time appeared to know little about this trouble.

He was put to bed for a year. There I was with two school children and a baby only two months old.

I was a great one for knowing the why of everything, and now I found this situation of my husband's illness no exception.

There were bound to be reasons, cures, even preventatives. Begging the doctors for information would get me nowhere for I already realized they were in a quandary. What I sought was the *real* answer, the simple method Nature had given us in the beginning.

So rewarding and fascinating was the knowledge gradually acquired that I never became sated, searching always, learning, applying them for my husband.

Through proper diet and mild exercise, he slowly overcame his bad heart and lived for many years.

How Author Reclaimed Youthfulness

By the time I was in my middle 40's, I began to realize that my youthful face was showing fine lines. My skin was a bit flabby. I did not feel the usual litheness in my body, and again I undertook to meet this challenge of oncoming old age. I began a system of exercise and was quite satisfied with the results until one day I met a woman hailing from Arizona, who told me of this system of reflex massage on feet and palms. She gave me a treatment, and I was amazed at how good I felt when she was finished. Not only was I revitalized, but my feet felt as though I walked on a cushion of air.

Not comprehending at first that this massage could be added to the knowledge I already had rather than being a thing apart, I gave much thought to whether or not I should pursue it in place of exercise, diet, and the other programs I had acquired through the years.

I felt I had found the answer about foot massage when I remembered all the passages in the Bible which had to do with the anointing of the feet.

Limitless Applications of Reflexology

The practice of *reflexology* is one of Nature's ways. It stimulates sick glands, and enables them to return to a healthy state.

Kidneys, Ovaries, and Hemorrhoids Healed

A friend had suffered for years with a kidney ailment, and had an ovary so diseased that she was scarcely able to hang laundry on her line. Three treatments relieved her of her symptoms, and when the course was finished, she also admitted to troublesome hemorrhoids which no longer plagued her (which was an extra bonus of the reflex treatments).

Epileptic Seizures

A woman brought her boy to me, telling me he had been subject to epileptic seizures since he was nine years old. He was then having as many as 27 spells a night at the age of 24.

The tender spots in his feet were many, denoting the condition of the main glands. This profusion made it difficult to decide which glands were causing his seizures. However, one treatment lessened his spells to one that night.

A few more treatments and he was able to discard most of his medication and had about an average of one seizure a week. The tenderness had left the bottoms of his feet and his foot massage treatments were reduced from every other day to one a week.

One sore spot remained which was located up under the big toe, a reflex to the parathyroid gland. "The doctors believe that is the root of his trouble," his mother declared, "but they could only give him medicine for it." Nevertheless, he had found the road to health.

From Heart Weakness to Rejuvenation

In the earlier years of my giving treatments in massage, a woman in her late 60's was brought to me. She had been in bed for three months, her heart presumably bad. She was helped up the steps and was breathing with difficulty. Her trembling hands denoted how nervous she was.

At that time, I had little experience in handling a heart patient and I undertook it with considerable care.

But I need not have been overly concerned, for my patient grew calm. She no longer panted. Her hands lay calmly in her lap.

She came to me every other day for a week, at the end of which time she was in good spirits, walking spryly up the steps without help.

Her treatments lessened to one a week, and as I worked on her feet, she would tell me of the miraculous changes throughout her body. The woman was actually going through a period of rejuvenation. Her sense of smell had been dulled and now she was able to gather in odors. Her sense of taste had been practically gone and now she enjoyed her food again.

The woman began to walk in her garden; then she was able to take the bus downtown shopping.

I found myself warning her, for the heart, being a muscle, had to have time to build back its strength. It was weak from not doing its proper share of work.

Some four years thereafter, I chanced to meet the woman's daughter and inquired about my former patient.

"Mother goes all around the country by bus, visiting relatives, having a delightful time," she told me.

Reflexology Benefits for Older People

Foot massage is especially good for elderly people for it rejuvenates the entire body, giving new life to the glands and cells. The blood flow has slowed over the years. Naturally, glands and cells become sluggish. Stimulating a new flow of blood to these tired places brings new life, clears glands and cells of accumulated poisons.

Cataracts of the Eyes

An elderly woman with cataracts came to me. I could not give her any encouragement that my treatments would give her any relief from this ailment, but she insisted that I try. Her husband brought her 200 miles once a week to see me. She had not made many such journeys until her near-blindness had been sufficiently overcome that she could read the advertisements on the signboards enroute. She no longer must be led into my office. She was able to see the denomination of the paper money she handled.

Female Disorders

An acquaintance was troubled with female disorders, and although she was only in her 30's her doctor had reserved a room for her in the hospital and she had arranged to have a hysterectomy. The doctor was primarily a surgeon, and I urged this woman to check with another doctor before she submitted to surgery.

She visited a doctor in an adjacent town, one specializing in disorders of women, and he declared her needs were only for minor surgery, so slight it could be taken care of in a doctor's office. "I suggest you have one more examination," he said, "since I am not practicing in your hometown and am a stranger to you."

The third doctor said she had ulcers and put her on an ulcer diet. About a month later, she called me and said she was very sick.

When I reached her home, I was alarmed. The woman had pulled off all her clothing. She lay on the couch gasping and writhing. I started on her foot massage and she began to grow more quiet.

Finally I was able to talk with her. She said she kept having these spells and was so terribly sick she was sure she was dying.

I had been home no longer than ten minutes when she summoned me to return. The second treatment brought relief again. When I reached home after this second trip, I consulted with my own doctor. I did not want to get involved with a serious heart condition, although there was no indication of it in the reflexes of her feet. He said he would make a house call and check.

The woman's heart was perfect. She had no high blood pressure. "I have no idea what is causing these spells," he declared. "Perhaps if she had been having one when I was there ... "

He reasoned that the only cause of such pain would be from an ulcer healing, if it were an exceedingly large one.

"You are coming home with me," I told her, and so I gathered her up along with her children and took them to my house. We had not been there more than a few minutes when she moaned that another attack was coming on.

Immediately I got busy on her feet, and by now I believed I knew the seat of her troubles. She needed something done for the liver and gallbladder. I massaged the reflexes governing these organs and was rewarded with a deep sigh. She closed her eyes and murmured weakly, "It is as if a huge blanket of pain had been lifted from me."

"You go to my doctor tomorrow," I suggested, "and tell him you believe your trouble is in the region of your liver and gallbladder. Avoid telling him why you believe this."

He sent her to the hospital for tests and x-rays, and these showed this to be true. The woman had gallstones, and surgery removed 13 of good size.

My doctor knew of my work and never tried to interfere with my doing it. In fact, there was another doctor in a small, neighboring town who always sent for a woman who was a reflex massager to solve puzzling cases which he could not diagnose.

Reflexology for Pets

My story of reflex massage and its individual cases would be something less than complete were I to omit the story of Inky, our little Pomeranian dog. This is a breed subject to asthma attacks. Inky, three years old, had an alarming attack of it one Sunday when we had guests. I kept rubbing his throat, giving him something to inhale to aid him in his breathing.

His difficulties did not lessen after we retired, he was in such discomfort that the family was kept awake by his attempts to breathe. Finally, I brought him to my side of the bed, rolled him over on his back, and began to massage his feet.

Certainly I had not the slightest notion where to rub a dog's foot to ease him of his asthma. With great care I massaged each pad of each toe, then the center large pad.

Five minutes of this and he quit his panic-stricken struggle to breathe. I discovered the small extra toe high up on the foot was the most tender spot.

All four feet thus treated, he relaxed and I fell asleep. I was awakened later in the night by his wheezing, but this time it was not as loud. When I called him to the bed from his own blanket in the room, he came readily, lying on his back, feet upturned for a second treatment!

Almost at once his breathing became easier and when I drifted off to sleep the second time, my little dog patient was slumbering also.

For all the rest of the years our pet was with us, he had few asthma attacks and when he did, the reflex massage quickly relieved him.

CHAPTER 4

Effective Reflex Massage Techniques

One excellent way to massage reflexes naturally is to follow the course of those who dwelt upon the earth many centuries ago. Remove your shoes and stockings and go about barefooted every chance you get.

I have influenced many of my neighbors to adopt this habit of removing footwear to work in the garden or to go across the street to visit a neighbor.

The Ideal Environment

The ideal environment, of course, is in the great outdoors. Get out in the country as often as possible. Walk on the bare earth. Walk on rocks and sticks as Nature intended that man should do. Be sure that the feet are *bare* so the electrical vibrations of the earth can be absorbed into the body, stimulating every living cell to renewed life and vitality.

Whenever one hunts or fishes, when he is in the mountains, at the seashore, playing golf, he should go without footwear as much as possible.

It is wise to hunt for rocks deliberately, walking on them. Hurt? Of course it will, especially if the walker has some sluggish, diseased parts of his body or sick cells in need of a fresh supply of blood.

The rocks will hunt out these reflexes, massaging them, breaking

21

up the crystals, allowing blood to flow freely again, washing away sluggishness and poisons.

Did you ever notice how quickly water freshens when good water is poured into muddy water? Never forget that good circulation is the essence of healthful life. Stagnation leads to untimely death. Just as a pond would soon become filled with algae and moss, eventually forming a hard crust, so will one's bloodstream, if a free, satisfactory circulation of blood is denied the cells and glands of all parts of the body.

Children should be encouraged to remove shoes and stockings. Plans should be made for trips to the mountains or out in the country. The entire family needs to walk over rough terrain, never avoiding sticks and stones. This can be turned into a game, the winner being the one who has come upon the most of these natural massagers!

But let us presume that there will be families who, for one reason or another, are not able to get out in the country. How can they give themselves a massage without the aid of Nature?

There is a device now on the market which is called the "Reflex Massager." It can be used conveniently in the privacy of one's own home. It can be used while the user is otherwise occupied, for it can be placed on the floor while one is standing or sitting. (See Fig. 4)

The principle of the massager is the same as that of the sticks and stones, only it can be used on the precise place it is needed for best results.

Along with the Reflex Massager is a chart explaining in detail where each reflex is in the feet and hands, which correspond with important glands and organs in the body. It is possible to decide which parts of the body need stimulating by massaging the reflexes in the feet.

It is well to be aware that the kidneys will invariably need attention, for the poison released from dealing with any other part of the body through reflexology will put extra labor on the kidneys. The kidneys comprise the filter system of the body and are to be stimulated last so they will be in condition for this extra burden put upon them.

The first few times the Reflex Massager is used, the treatment should be cautiously done. Too much poison flowing into the

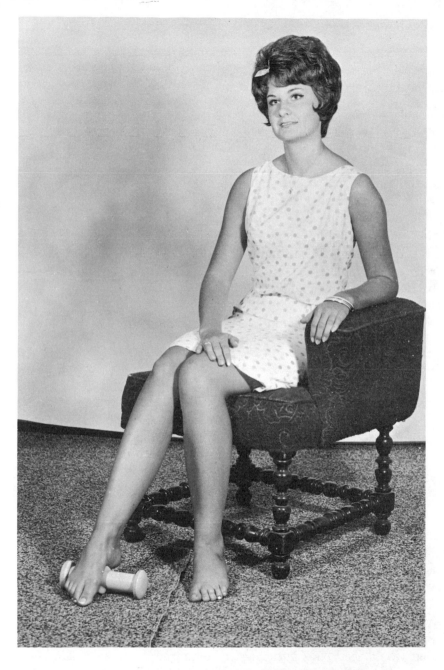

Fig. 4. Position for using the Reflex Massager.

system at once can result in making one feel ill.

Length of Reflexology Treatment

This early treatment should not extend over, probably, ten minutes, and every other day for the first week.

The resulting discomfort would do no harm, but it could prove discouraging and result in failure to continue the treatments. The general good will be inevitable, relaxing the nerves, stimulating veins, endocrine glands, and aiding the diaphragm.

It can be appreciated that one should first study the charts thoroughly, learning where the reflexes are in the bottoms of the feet, thus enabling him to diagnose his own illnesses. By becoming efficient in massaging the feet, locating tender spots, and referring to the charts, he will know what gland in his body is in special need of stimulation.

Reflex massage is the natural way back to health.

Location of Reflexes

So little appears to be known, generally, concerning reflexes. These reflexes are not *in* the skin, but *under* it. Some are in an area as large as a lima bean. Others are no bigger than the head of a pin, so one must press sufficiently hard to find them. Sometimes considerable searching is involved at first.

How to Locate Reflexes

The reflexes can aptly be termed "buttons," for massaging them is not unlike pressing a button. Let us presume you did not feel well, but you did not know exactly where you felt ill. You would get out your massager, or, not having one, use your fingers or even a rubber pencil eraser. You would press gently, but firmly, on the bottom of one foot, using a rotating motion, hunting for the button that would send back a message of tenderness or actual pain. This would indicate a congested area. A full flow of life-giving blood is being denied this spot.

You refer to your charts as set out previously to discover what part of the body is sending you this summons for help. Massage the button for a few seconds. Don't be alarmed by the pain of it, and don't massage with such force that the tiny capillaries may be injured.

It will be a revelation when you realize how Nature aids you in knowing where to massage, and how hard to massage if you approach the treatment gradually.

The entire foot should be massaged in order not to miss any of the buttons waiting to give out distress signals. Each time one such button is located, it is to receive a brief, gentle, and thorough massage.

Go to the other foot and repeat the procedure. Never be guilty of taking only half a treatment.

Suppose an electrician came and repaired one socket in your home which had become corroded, but along the line there were other places where the cord was frayed and suffering from corrosion. His first repairs might give electricity to a part of your home, but perhaps the important rooms might still be in darkness.

Another example is the battery of your car. If corrosion has settled on the cable, there will be no spark. When the corrosion is broken loose and sanded off, the cable can make a direct contact and the car comes to life. There is spark where needed, *unless* other places in the cable are similarly afflicted.

So it is, when you find a *corroded button* in the bottom of your foot. Start massaging it, around and around, or back and forth, aware that you are wearing away the corrosion which has slowed the circulation to a certain portion of your body, making it impossible to work as perfectly as it was made to do.

When using the Reflex Massager on the floor, it will be easy to press the buttons that are tender. It also should be easy to find the buttons which are giving you trouble.

The hand massager of the Rollo type is excellent for this. (See Fig. 5.)

Palm Reflexes

These same reflexes found in the bottom of the feet are also to be found in the palms of the hands, but since hands do such a great amount of work, the palm reflexes can be worked out generally in

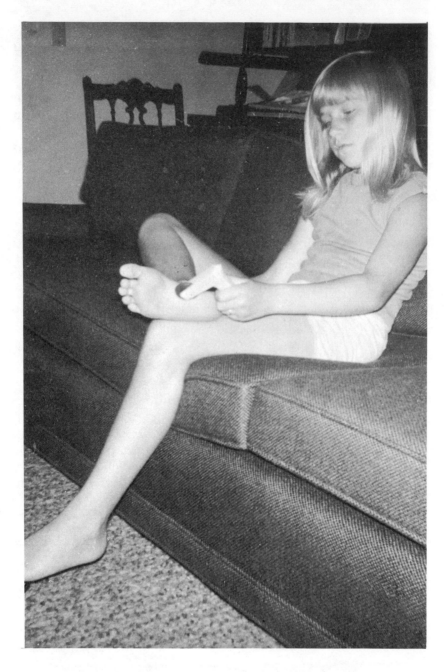

Fig. 5. The simplicity of using the Rollo Reflex Massager.

the day's usual routine.

If one is especially inactive, never using his hands to grip with or pick up objects, the buttons under the skin of the palms must be massaged too. The Rollo Massager is especially efficient here. Lacking one, the thumb of the opposite hand can do much to probe for tender buttons in need of massage, as well as do a fairly good job of massaging, especially on the fingers.

The fact that the feet hold us upright, sustain our weight, and experience an increased amount of pressure, make their reflex centers more important for massaging.

Reflex Remote Control

A pressure on a certain button in the foot can result in an odd tingling sensation in quite another part of the body, and you will know that the reflex button has connected with this remote part. You then have proof that the healing message of the reflex is getting through to the source of trouble.

Sometimes the tingling will be in a part of the body where you least expect it, and this is encouraging. You have discovered a life-giving current of health! It is this reward which makes reflex massage of such value. It covers all parts of the body and brings them under control. It keeps any corrosion from forming and causing trouble at a later time.

The Rollo Massager is good for working on the upper parts of the feet, and the legs.

Having located a tender spot, be sure that the tenderness remains apparent as you continue the treatment. If it is tender in the first instant of contact, then is not tender, you may be sure you have either gotten off the spot or are not pressing as hard on it as you should be.

Basic Points to Bear in Mind

Avoid massaging in one place very long, especially at first. Go from one sore spot to another, rotating. Often, when you come back to an earlier-treated spot, you will find that much of the tenderness has already left, even completely vanished.

You will know from your charts that it is in the center of the foot where the kidneys are treated. Since so much does depend on them in this cleansing process, beware of overdoing the massage of this area. Give those important organs a chance to carry off the poisons without rushing this form of reflexology too quickly for best results.

If congestion is bad and of long standing, probably the massage of the foot should not be longer than five minutes per foot the first time. Skip a day, then massage perhaps ten minutes for each foot, and then only if you are able to detect less tenderness.

One must keep in mind that he has been a long time getting in the condition he now finds himself. He must give Nature a chance to correct this, although often the improvement is so rapid it does seem like a miracle.

It is wise to try to begin your foot massage at a time when you can go to bed right afterward, or at least enjoy a nap, for these massages *are* relaxing.

European Methods vs. Reflexology Massage

In Germany, there is a new method of treatment being used by two doctors who claim extraordinary success.

Doctor Ferdinand Huneke and his brother, Walter, use a healing method which is called *neural therapy*. They inject a local anaesthetic in certain parts of the body to bring about instant healing.

A recent health magazine article stated that the method of achieving this instant healing effect was through the nervous system; specifically, through the vegetative (autonomic) nervous system. Neural therapy deals with an unspecific stimulus type of treatment. A directed stimulus put into the right place is capable of inducing real healing through a lightning-quick change of the electrophysical state of the vegetative nerves, with accompanying instant freedom from pain and discomfort.

With neural therapy, doctors have to study the case history of the patient in order to find the pathological connections which induce healing. They study all previous illnesses that preceded the present trouble. This might be an old injury that left scars, an infection that was still present in a different part of the body.

It is claimed that the exhaustive searching back into a patient's past medical history opens up many questions for researchers in the field. This is, indeed, true, and nobody realizes it more than a person engaged in massaging the reflexes.

A neural therapist has to observe and ask questions. He needs great patience with his subject, who is not able to understand why an old, forgotten injury or sickness could, after many years, be responsible for an illness quite different.

Only an extensive case history makes the discovery of a connection possible in *neural therapy*. In reflex massage, we do not have to know about past injuries or illnesses. *They will show up in the tenderness of the reflexes in the bottoms of the feet.*

Reflex massage therapy compares with neural therapy in that instantaneous healing is not unknown in either of these two forms of treatment. This is so probably because the same electrophysical processes are employed in both therapies, although in a different and simpler way in reflexology.

Sometimes, after certain damages, the body does not manage to recuperate completely and regain its former condition. A permanent change remains in the tissues, and often this goes unrecognized. This is reflected in the electrophysical relationship of the tissues. A field of disturbance is thus created, from which faulty stimuli may be directed to any other part of the body or organism by the electrically structured vegetative nerves. It is very possible that any chronic disease may be triggered by a field of disturbance that can be in any part of the organism.

Scars as a Source of Body Disturbance

Scars, in particular, have proved to be a field of disturbance for a great number of disorders.

This brings us back to reflex massage! Used on the feet, it covers the body. If there is trouble from an old scar or from illness, the reflex to this complication is reached by massaging, even if its existence is unknown.

It is interesting to realize that an old scar on your leg could be causing the pain in your head! It is also equally gratifying to know that you have only to do a thorough job of foot massage and the rest will take care of itself.

CHAPTER 5

Reflex Massage of the Toes

There is no portion of your wonderfully constructed foot which does not have its part to play in this reflex massage. The foot offers a new, unique way to health through its reflex treatment. I shall give you a detailed account of how to apply the simple and natural method of massaging your own feet, to bring to yourself a new way to attain vibrant health.

You have now studied the charts and have a general idea of how each different part of your body has a corresponding reflex located some place on the feet, and where to locate these corresponding reflexes.

You have found a position in which you are comfortable and relaxed while reaching your feet easily (one at a time, of course). (See Fig. 6.)

You understand the gentle, deep, circular pressing motion that you must use to reach these reflexes in order to massage them correctly. If you don't reach the inner reflex button it will not be able to send a stimulation to the distressed part of the body, nor will you be able to break up the accumulated crystals in the capillaries.

Finding the Pituitary Reflex

You are ready for your first experience in the vitalizing, rejuvenating method the health-building field of reflexology offers

31

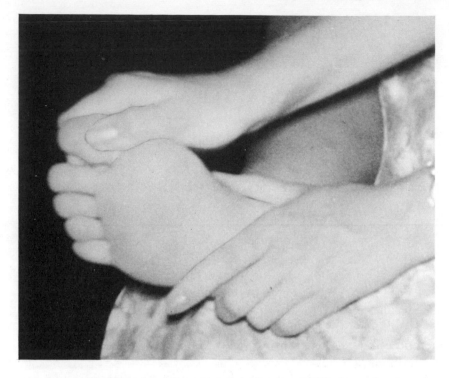

Fig. 6. Position for massaging the reflex to the pituitary gland.

you. You will now learn how to massage your own feet.

Take your left foot in your left hand and with the fingers of the right hand press the big toe gently all over. Do you feel any tender spots? If not, then press a little harder with a circular motion. This is just so you can get the feel of it.

We will start by massaging the pituitary reflex in the center of the big toe, since this is the most important gland that we have (See Fig. 7.)

Notice in the picture of the pituitary reflex how the instrument is pressed into the center of the pad on the big toe. I don't believe that you can find this reflex with the fingers unless it is extremely tender. Although the spot is no larger than the head of a pin, touching it in the act of massage is like sticking a pin in the toe. This is especially true with older people whose circulation to the pituitary has been cut down for many years.

It will be found that, by sending new stimulation to this gland in the young or old, there will be a new lease on life. Age is not always a factor. Many young people do not have as good a pituitary as someone older. In many, especially in men, the reflexes may be very deep and the pressure will have to be equally deep to reach them.

Here the small, hand Reflex Massager is especially good. If it is not available, try a pencil with a new eraser, or other like device. Now press the device into the soft pad of the big toe in the very center; keep pressing with a little, rotating motion. If you don't feel a sharp stab of pain, either you are not on it, or you are not pressing deeply enough. Be careful not to bruise the tender capillaries in the skin while doing this. When you feel a sharp pain, then you are on the reflex to the pituitary gland. Having found it, massage it with a gentle, circular motion — two or three seconds the first time.

Pineal Gland

You are also near the reflex to the pineal gland, which, as you can see in Charts 1 and 3, is located near the center of the brain; so the reflexes to the pineal would be located near the center of the big toe, just a tiny bit toward the second toe and a bit up toward the tip of the toe. Try finding this spot by the same method you used in locating the reflex to the pituitary gland. Massage it for a few seconds with a gentle, circular motion.

Now put your left foot on the floor and pick up the right foot in the same position you just used on the left, taking the right foot in the right hand and massaging the big toe with the fingers of the left hand. Next, take the massager and press it into the center of the pad of the big toe, working it around until you feel the sharp pain that tells you that you are pressing on the pituitary reflex. Massage it for a few seconds no matter how painful it is. Sometimes you only need to touch it two or three times the first time to get results. Then find the reflex to the pineal and massage as you did on the left foot. This also may be quite painful, but that is all the more reason it needs massaging. You will be amazed how quickly the soreness will work out of the reflexes to these two glands — sometimes in only two or three treatments.

Put your right foot back on the floor and lift the left foot back into position. Changing the legs often keeps them from becoming

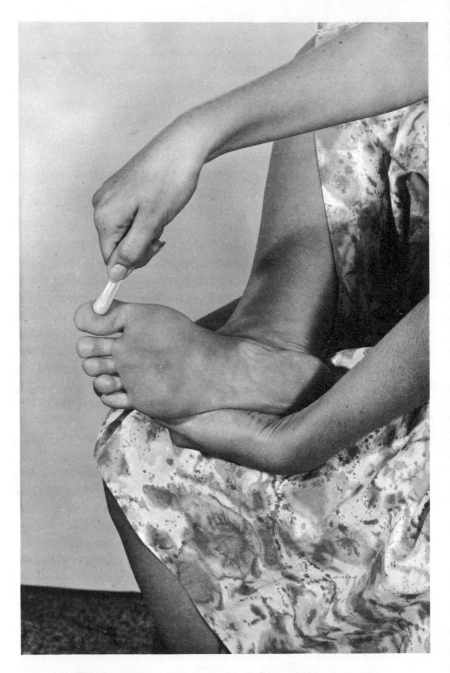

Fig. 7. Position for massaging the reflexes in the big
toe, with the hand Reflex Massager.

too cramped by holding them in one position too long. After awhile the muscles will become accustomed to these positions and you will not need to change legs as often. (Study the chapters on the glands.)

Further Techniques with Big Toe

Let's continue to work on the big toe. Remember, the left foot represents the left side of the body, so when we massage the big toe of the left foot we are contacting the reflexes to the left side of the head. Take the big toe in the fingers of the right hand and massage it with a pressing, rotating motion covering the whole toe. You will probably find several tender spots at first; massage them gently for a few seconds. Notice in Fig. 8 on how to massage the reflexes on the top of the big toe where the thumb is pressing just below the nail; these reflexes would generally stimulate the back of the head and the teeth. This is the area that is massaged in case of a stroke.

The top side of the toe may be pressed in various places until a tender spot is found which may be the reflex to the part of the brain containing the clot causing the stroke. A general coverage of the whole toe is the surest method of massage for the best results. (See Fig. 8.)

On the inside of the large toe, you may come upon a very tender spot. This is a reflex to the outer side of the head or brain. Be sure that it is well massaged until all tenderness is gone, which is possible in many cases in one treatment.

As we move on down the toe toward the foot we find the reflexes on the top of the toe to be the reflexes to the back of the neck. Notice here how the bones of the big toe connect to those of the arch of the foot, and how they resemble the bones of the spine, which Chart 1 illustrates. The inside of the big toe next to the second toe will have the reflexes to the outer side of the neck, while the outside of the big toe will contain those to the center of the neck.

Throat and Tonsil Reflexes

The bottom or underside of the big toe where it fastens onto the foot has the reflexes to the tonsils and throat. In case of sore

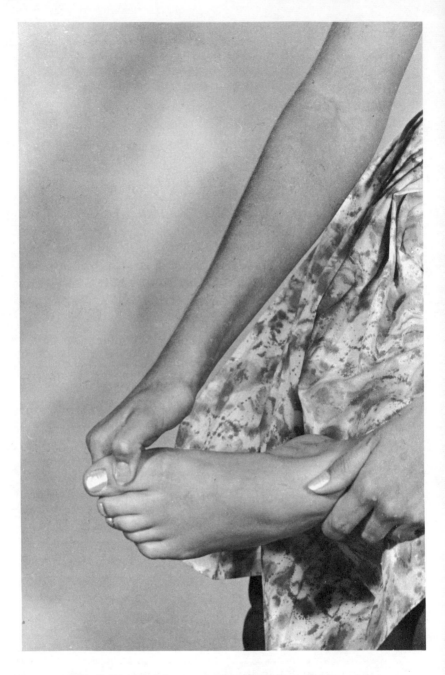

Fig. 8. Position for massaging the reflexes on top of the big toe.

throat, you will find this very tender. Massage just under the pad of the big toe down to where the toe fastens onto the foot. You will find a tender spot in this area and can quickly relieve the throat trouble by massaging these reflexes.

Case of Sore Throat Healed

Recently a neighbor came to me saying her three-year-old son was suffering with a sore throat. His fever was very high. Returning home with her, I rubbed the reflexes to the throat (the underside of the big toe). And because of the fever, I also massaged the reflexes to the pituitary gland, in the center of the big toe. Later in the day, I saw him out playing in the snow!

Children are the most willing subjects for massage. They appear to crave it, instinct prompting them to indulge in the treatment. Many whom I know are given to urging their mothers to call me instead of a doctor when they are ill.

This all sums up to the fact that if there is tenderness anywhere on the big toe, there is tension and congestion which must be released in the interest of good health.

Headaches and Eye Weakness

Tension in the neck causes many headaches and eye weaknesses. So, after massaging the entire big toe, relax this neck area by taking the big toe in the fingers and rotating it in a circular motion — first to the left, then to the right, around and around, until it feels loose.

This may take a few treatments, but the results will be especially satisfying. It is the same as though someone took your head in his hands and gently rotated it in a similar manner, only this method of working through the big toe would give better results.

If your leg feels tired, you had better change positions again and work on the toe of the right foot before we go on to the massaging of the next toes.

Now that you have massaged both big toes, let's move on to the toe next to the big one. Between these two toes, close to where they are fastened onto the foot, more at the base of the second toe, there is a reflex to some part of the head which stops many headaches. Often a tenderness here is noticed on only one foot, but it is a rewarding place to get relief from a headache, in many cases when nothing else will help. If you cannot find a tender spot here, and your headache is still throbbing, try other spots on the toes and between them also. I have never failed to relieve a headache with reflex massage, even in cases of migraine and other factors.

Headaches are frequently caused by the upset of some organ, such as the stomach or liver, in which case the reflex to the organ should be worked on in conjunction with the toes.

Reflexes of the Eyes

At the bottom of the second toe and the one next to it, you will find the reflexes to the eyes. (See Chart 1 and also the illustration in Fig. 9.)

To massage these reflexes, you hold the foot in position and press with a rolling motion just under these two toes. This is usually easy to do with your fingers, but in some cases you may find it more rewarding to use the Reflex Massager or a like device. Press and roll this area, searching for tender spots, and when you find them, massage each one for a few seconds. Many different cases of near blindness have been helped by the massaging of the reflexes in the feet. Not only are the direct eye reflexes responsible for eye disorders, but there are taut nerves in the back of the neck which cause a normal blood supply to the head and eyes to be cut off. Also, remember that when there is an abnormal condition of the eyes, the functioning of the kidneys appears to be a contributing factor in the case. Therefore, massaging of the kidney and adrenal reflexes is important, too.

Ear Reflexes

Still holding the foot in the same position, let's go to the reflexes of the ears, which are in a similar position to the eye reflexes, only just under the next two toes, the fourth and fifth. (See Chart 1.) We will massage these reflexes just as we did for the eyes. Keep in mind

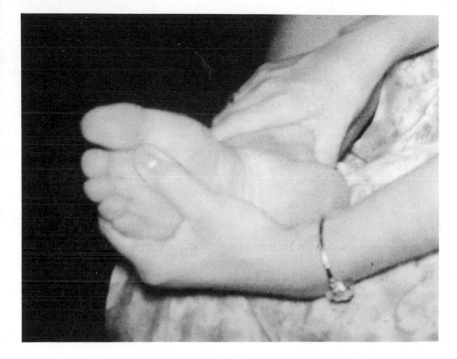

**Fig. 9. Position for massaging the reflexes for head-
ache, eyes, ears, and sinuses.**

that the right foot governs the right ear; the left foot, the left ear.

The taut nerves of the neck could have the same abnormal effect on the ears as they do on the eyes.

Forever be aware that any tenderness needs appropriate massage. This indicates that somewhere there is tension which needs release, or congestion which prevents the blood from flowing freely into some area.

Sinus Reflexes

Now let us go back to the position of the reflexes of the eyes and ears. You will find by dropping down into the foot just a tiny bit below the eye and ear reflexes, the reflexes to the sinuses. You will massage them in the same manner that you massage the reflexes of the eyes and ears. There is one spot, especially between the second and third toes, that seems to have a very definite reflex to the sinuses. After you find the right tender spot in this area, you may massage this reflex for several minutes, or until you can feel the congestion of the sinuses loosening up.

Rub the tips of each toe with the Reflex Massager or the thumbnail, by rolling either one across the top of each toe just in front of the nail. This also tends to relieve sinus congestion. Now, take each toe, one at a time, and give it two or three light twists and rolls for relaxing.

CHAPTER 6

Reflex Techniques for the Spine

The spine's importance to general health is familiar to all practitioners. Osteopathic and chiropractic doctors understand that the greater part of one's well-being depends on the condition of the spine. To massage the reflexes of the back or spine is to relax the muscle tension surrounding any vertebra that is not in perfect and healthful alignment.

You have studied the position of the spine and its reflexes in Chart 1. Look at Fig. 10 on massaging the spine reflexes. Notice how the thumb of the right hand is pressing into the center of the instep of the right foot! This is where the reflex to the spine is located, and the spot that the thumb is pressing would be a reflex to about the center of the back or the waistline.

Have your foot up in position. Now take the large toe, beginning just at the bottom of it. Remember the big toe represents the head and the neck. Now, feel just below the big toe for the first vertebra of the spine reflex. Follow these bones on down the foot with the fingers and notice how they resemble the bones in your back.

Relief of Back Tensions or Pain

If there is pain or tension in the upper part of the back, as between the shoulders or around the neck, look for tenderness just below the large toe. If there is backache in the center of the back, then look for tenderness in the middle of the foot, around the waistline. If you have lower back trouble, then follow the inner side

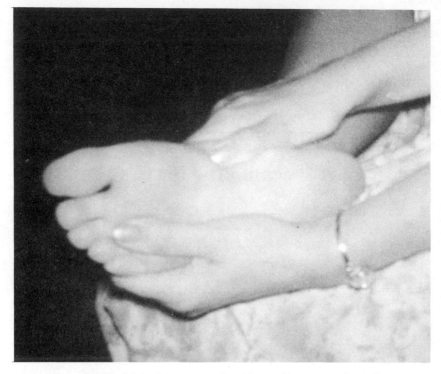

Fig. 10. Position for massaging the reflexes to the spine.

of the foot down to the heel. Using the pressing, rolling motion along these bones in the foot, search out the tender spots with the fingers.

Press slightly in and under the bones of the foot, especially in the area just above the heel, which is the lower lumbar region, shown in Chart 1.

The whole spinal column is located in the exact center of the body, so the reflexes will cover the entire area of the inside of each foot, lengthwise, from the toe to the heel.

Notice in the picture on the massage of the bladder reflex (Fig. 17 on page 103), how close it is to the reflex of the lower lumbar region. By just moving the thumb a little bit toward the heel you will be on the reflex to the lower lumbar region, and the end of the spine or tailbone.

Keep this picture in mind and you will have no trouble locating a weakness in the back, by the location of the tenderness on the inside of the foot. When this tenderness is located, massage it gently at first, as it may be extremely tender. As you massage this tenderness out, by working on the reflexes, you are causing a definite relaxing effect on the spine. If there is an injury to the spine, or it is in any way out of alignment, you will find that as you relax the tension in the spinal reflex, your muscles will cease to contract. Thus in Nature's own natural way the vertebra will be able to return to its natural position, restoring once again the proper circulation.

Remember when working on the spinal reflexes that every part of your body receives its nerve supply from some part of the spine. An impinged nerve tightening the muscles, thus causing abnormal tension, is the cause of a big majority of our ailments.

Reflexes for Full Length of Spine

It is wise to massage the reflexes for the full length of the spine at least a minute or two each time the feet are massaged. Thus tension on the spinal column and the whole spine area is relaxed, and muscles cease to contract. The spinal vertebrae will become perfectly aligned and circulation will be as Nature intended it.

Case Histories of Spinal Healings

Following are a couple of cases which prove beyond a doubt the therapeutic value of reflex massage for the spine.

A woman went skating with her children, and had a very bad fall, landing on the end of her spine. She called me the next day and said she had called a bone specialist to take x-rays but she was in much pain. Would I please come over and see if I could bring her some relief until she could get to the doctor, as it would be two days before she could see him? I went to her house and upon massaging her feet found severe tenderness in the lower lumbar region, which I proceeded to massage very gently. The full length of the foot on the spinal area was affected to some degree, but the lower lumbar reflex was so sensitive that I could barely touch it at first. I changed from one foot to the other often, though I found the reflex on the right foot much more tender than the reflex on the left one, indicating that she had injured the right side of the spine. After about a half hour of massaging the spine reflexes the pain subsided, and she was able to get up and do her work. She felt so much better that she called the bone specialist and canceled her appointment. I urged her to go to a doctor for an examination but she never did. She took a few more treatments from me, and although her back was sore for quite a while after her accident, she fully recovered and never did go to a doctor. That was about ten years ago.

The Author's Experience

The second case involves myself. I was fishing in a small stream and as I stepped on a rock it turned with me. I quickly threw my weight onto another rock which also turned under my foot, throwing me off balance and into the stream. I landed on my back on a rock in the shallow water. The pain was so severe that I think I passed out for a second, the cold water rushing over my face reviving me. I crawled out onto the bank and lay there awhile, but forced myself to get up, as I did not want to lie there long enough to become too stiff to walk. It was over a mile to the car, and I had to drive 70 miles over mountainous roads to get home.

I suffered terrible pain all night after arriving home. The next day I had to paint my living room as I was moving into a new house. The room was empty except for a ladder. Every time I tried to climb the ladder to paint the ceiling I was in such pain I had to quit. I hadn't been studying reflex massage very long at this time, but I sat down in the middle of the floor and took one of my feet in my hands. I had struck my back about 3 inches above the waistline when I fell on the rock, so I felt along the inside of my foot up just a little from the center and there I found a spot so tender that it made tears come to my eyes to touch it. I knew I had the right spot so I persisted with a gentle massage, first on one foot, then on the other, until I got some of the soreness worked out. In my case, as in the case of my friend who hurt her back, most of the tenderness was in one foot. After about 20 minutes of massage, a lot of the soreness had been worked out. To my own amazement, when I got up my back was so improved that I was able to finish painting the ceiling and walls of the room, which was quite large. The pain in my back never returned, though it was a little sore for about ten days.

Unlimited Massage Time for the Back

The reflexes of the back and other bone areas may be massaged for an unlimited time, unlike the glands where time must be limited to a few seconds for the first few treatments. Following is a most interesting case history on a very involved situation concerning the back and related disorders.

Case History of a Serious Back Situation and Its Healing

At a dance that I was attending I was introduced to a man whom I thought at the time was a hunchback. I thought what a shame for such a nice looking man to be so deformed. He stood slumped over with a big bulge standing out along his back and shoulders. I found him to be quite a good dancer and later became better acquainted with him.

I learned that he had suffered family tragedies which had made him quite despondent. I got around to telling him about the reflexology treatments I gave and how they proved to be doing such amazing things for those who tried them. He had never heard of them before and was intensely interested. He said he had several health problems and would like to try the reflexology treatments.

He made an appointment to come to the office in a few days. When he arrived and I had him seated comfortably in the chair, I learned that besides having a bad back he suffered from several other complaints. All of the reflexes were quite tender, and as I worked down to the stomach reflex under the area of the reflexes to the thyroid, I noticed that it was exceptionally sensitive to the touch. "Do you have stomach trouble?", I asked him. "I have an ulcer," he replied. As I massaged on down the foot I found that the kidneys were also very tender. He admitted to having spells of trouble with what he had suspected to have been caused by his kidneys. As I massaged the liver reflex under the little toe area on the right foot and found it very sore, I went to the reflexes of the colon and found them just as tender as the ones to the liver. I asked him if he had any trouble with constipation and his reply to that was, "I have been constipated all of my life. I know you can't help that, it's just part of me." I just said, "Wait and see." Then as my fingers moved down to the ankles, I learned that he had a lot of tenderness in the reflexes to the prostate gland. I asked him if he

had known of a weakness there. He said no, that he hadn't. I asked
if he had to get up nights, and he said yes, several times, and he
couldn't understand it because when he got to the bathroom he
didn't seem to have to go as bad as he had thought. So he laid the
blame to nerves.

Men usually become quite upset when you mention that there
might be a weakness in the prostate gland. Reflexology seems to
bring new life to the prostate through added circulation and a
renewal of life forces. These are enabled to get through and disperse
the congestion that has started to build up in this gland. I have never
treated a case of prostate trouble that didn't receive great benefit
from the massaging of the reflex to it.

I was able to assure my patient that his prostate condition was
not serious and he would find that he would have no more trouble
of that kind within a few days. It is amazing how quickly the
prostate responds when the reflexes under the ankles on the inside
of the feet are massaged.

As I continued to work on the feet of my patient I also found
that he was affected with hay fever and sinus. The poor man has
really got himself out of harmony with the universe, I thought, as I
massaged each reflex gently. He was the type that would suffer in
silence and it was hard to know how hard to press without causing
undue pain the first time. It is unnecessary to press hard initially
because the reflexes will become less tender with each treatment
after the third treatment, unless we come up against something that
is chronic or cannot be helped with reflex massage alone.

I knew that I was going to find quite a reaction when I started on
the back reflexes, so I had left this until the last. All of the area
below the big toe following the bone on the inside of the foot down
to about the center of the foot was so sore that it was even more
than he could stand without flinching. He said that he had been
hurt when in the service, but that nothing was done about it
because it was just before they shipped out to go overseas in World
War II, and so many of the boys were faking illnesses and injuries
to keep from going over to fight. He had suffered off and on with it
ever since, and as he grew older it became worse. At times he
would be in such pain when he tried to get out of bed in the morning
that he couldn't move. Sometimes he would lie in agony for as long
as three weeks. He had gone to all kinds of doctors.

They all agreed that he had a very bad spine but did not know what to do unless they operated on it. He was thinking seriously of resorting to that as a last hope of relief.

I tried to build his hopes up by telling him of the many cases of back troubles I had helped with reflex massage.

This man had both mental and physical problems that would have made many men give up all hope a long time ago. He had heavy worries and a broken heart from the loss of his family, which were in part responsible for some of his physical complaints, but not the back. His legs had started to go numb at times and he had a dead feeling in part of his leg that he had noticed ever since he was first injured in the Navy.

After taking several treatments, my patient had recovered beyond his belief. All signs of the prostate trouble vanished after the second treatment, and he said he slept all night without moving. In fact, he slept at every opportunity he had for the next month. It seemed that he just couldn't get enough sleep, he said. I told him that it was his body healing, since all of its functions had been reawakened by the life forces and a new surge of circulation throughout his whole system. His body mechanisms were literally turned loose by Nature after the reflexes were massaged enough to give her a chance to go to work as she was intended to.

It was interesting to watch the symptoms of each illness the reflexes had shown him to have disappear one by one. As his nerves grew calm and his mental depression vanished like a mist, he became more cheerful and the ulcer disappeared. He had no more kidney attacks, and for the first time that he could remember he was free of constipation and has never been bothered with it since.

He stopped having headaches, and as the muscles in the back started to relax from massaging the reflexes to it, he was able to stand straighter every day. He was not deformed at all; he had just given the appearance of a hunchback because he was pulled forward and over by pain and tight muscles. Of course, the injured spine is still as it was, but he very seldom has any pain, and never any attacks that lay him up as they used to.

That has been quite a few years ago and none of his old symptoms has returned. I know this is a fact because I did such a good job of returning this particular man to perfect health with reflex massage that I married him!

CHAPTER 7

Massage of Thyroid Gland Reflexes

We are now ready to massage the reflexes to the thyroid gland. Study the basic charts in the beginning of this book and see where in the body the thyroid is located, then take a look at Fig. 11 showing the thyroid reflexes being massaged.

The right foot is being held by the left hand, and the right hand is used for the massage. Notice how the thumb is pressed under the bone of the pad just under the big toe, inside the large toe bone, toward the center of the foot.

Start at the base of the big toe with the thumb pressing in under the bone as much as possible. Use a rolling motion and follow the bone down to the inside edge of the foot, as shown in Fig. 11. Massage along this pad covering the toe bone with the thumb or massager. If using the massager, roll the sharp edge back and forth as much under the bone as possible.

This is another endocrine gland and extremely important to one's well-being and will be dealt with in another chapter.

Press along this pad until you hit the reflex to the thyroid. You will experience a sharp pain, and the whole area may be quite tender, with the pain very pronounced at first, but eventually the crystals will be broken loose and washed away by the released bloodstream. You will notice the pain becoming less and less.

Sometimes you will have to dig quite deeply to reach this reflex. It is especially deep on some men.

This important hormone-producing gland is not to be neglected. Often one is able to feel this crunching of accumulated crystals as one massages over them.

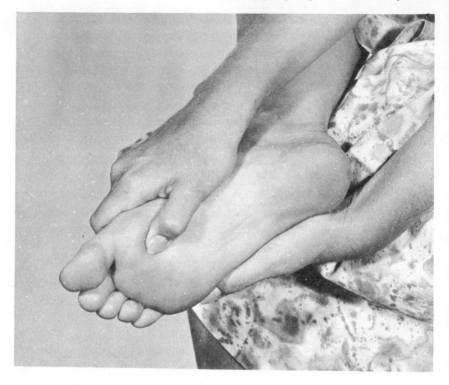

Fig. 11. Position for massaging the reflexes to the thyroid gland.

The Importance of the Thyroid

Remember the importance of the thyroid gland when you are massaging the reflexes to it. Any derangement of this gland may affect the other glands, especially the pituitary and the adrenals. The hormones sent into the bloodstream by the thyroid gland are very important for breaking down the waste products of the body. Its malfunction can be the starting point for obesity, overweight, etc. It can also cause profound internal changes, high blood pressure, and kidney troubles. Many criminals and inmates of mental institutions may be victims of a thyroid deficiency.

There are substitutes for glandular hormones, to temporarily provide relief, such as ACTH, cortisone, insulin, etc. However, you can restore the functioning of your glands to normal so Nature can produce her own glandular secretions by massaging the reflexes to each one of these glands faithfully until they have returned to normal. If you are one of those people who feel as though you were born tired, find your mentality becoming dull, feel inattentive, and sleepy, you may need the hormone secretion produced by the thyroid gland to supply your body with the fuel and energy to wake you up and give you that lift that you need. Massage the reflex to the thyroid, and enable it to produce its own normal secretion according to Nature's plan.

Reflexes of the Parathyroids

If you will look again at Chart 3 of the endocrine glands at the beginning of the book, you will notice the location of the tiny parathyroid glands. There are two on each side of the thyroid and they lie just in back of the lobes. You can easily see that you will use the same position and the same location to massage these tiny but very important glands. You will have to press in a little deeper than you do for the thyroid, and since they are so small, you will have to use your own judgment in massaging them. Generally, the parathyroids will get enough benefit from the massaging of the thyroid, unless there is a definite congestion within them.

This is the gland that is responsible for your poise and tranquility, besides many other important body functions which I will explain further in another chapter.

Use of the massager will probably be needed to reach the reflexes of the parathyroids to enable you to press back in behind the thyroid reflexes. Be very careful not to bruise the tissue or capillaries with the deep massage.

When you get through massaging the reflexes to the thyroid and parathyroid glands on the one foot, change positions and massage the opposite foot in the same manner.

CHAPTER 8

Reflexes to Lungs and Bronchial Tubes

Let's look again at Chart 2 to see the position of the lungs. Notice how they lie in the chest, and then note how the reflexes to the lungs are situated along the pads of the feet which lie below the toes, under the reflexes to the eyes and the ears. You will also notice that the lungs take up quite a large space in the chest area. Similarly the reflexes to the lungs take up quite an area on the foot. Remember, right foot, right lung; left foot, left lung.

The position to massage the lungs would be the same as you used to massage the thyroid (Fig. 11). Hold the right foot with the left hand and use the fingers of the right hand to massage along the reflexes to the lungs. Use a circular, rolling motion as you cover the whole pad under the toes. Use of the massager will make the massaging of this area easier, by rolling it across the foot, back and forth, and also up and down, so that the whole area may be well covered.

The trachea (windpipe) and lungs are parts of the respiratory system, which delivers oxygen to the blood. The lungs consist of millions of elastic membranous sacs which together can hold about as much air as a basketball. The lungs are constantly inflating and emptying in their crucial capacity as a medium of exchange. The lungs sustain life by unloading carbon dioxide and taking in oxygen carried by the blood to the cells. Oxygen unlocks the energy contained in the body's fuels. The body's trillions of cells require so much oxygen that we need about 30 times as much surface for its intake as our entire skin area covers. The lungs provide this surface

53

area (even though they weigh only about 2½ pounds on the average) and fit neatly within the chest cavity, due to the fact that their membranes fold over and over on themselves in pockets thinner than a sheet of paper.

Even the purest country air contains dust particles and bacteria. City air, of course, is additionally burdened with soot and exhaust fumes. As the air passes through the nose, some of its dust particles and bacteria drop off; others are trapped by tiny hairs or mucus. In the windpipe, most of the remaining bacteria in the air are intercepted by mucus.

The bronchi are two large tubes, one for each lung, leading off the trachea (or windpipe) like the limbs of a tree, which taper on down into smaller bronchi tubes to make a treelike formation within the lungs. You can see how disastrous it is for the body when a severe infection of these muscular bronchi results in destruction of the muscle necessary for contraction.

Reflex massage of the whole area of the lungs will benefit the bronchial tubes. You will hold the same position as when massaging the lung reflexes. Start the massage under the big toe, in the same place as the throat reflexes, so that you will be sure to cover the reflexes to the larynx (or vocal cords) at the top of the trachea (windpipe). With the thumb, you press into the soft area starting under the big toe and massage down to the pad under the toes. If there is any tenderness, massage it with a pressing, circular motion. If there is any indication of congestion in the lungs or the bronchials, then massage this area thoroughly. Even if you do not find tenderness, you may not be getting deep enough. But we know, where there is congestion, there is trouble; so massage it out.

Colds

While we are on the subject of the lungs, I want to mention the effects of colds. A cold is Nature's way of cleaning house; I mean eliminating the system of toxic acid. It is trying to rid the body of accumulated poisons, through the pores of the skin, and the mucous membrane in the head, nose, and sinuses. So do not massage the reflexes to the whole body when you have a cold. Remember, it is already overburdened with eliminating poisons, so just give Nature a little help instead of hindrance by massaging the toes and lung area, and including a very *short* massage of the kidney reflex. The pituitary reflex can be concentrated on in case of fever.

CHAPTER 9

How to Handle Stomach Reflexes

The stomach lies high in the abdomen, on the left side, nested up under the diaphragm and protected by the rib cage. In form it is kind of a pouch, about 10 inches long, with a diameter that depends on its contents. When full, it can stretch to hold as much as 2 quarts of food. When empty, it collapses on itself like a deflated balloon. Food materials take the same route along the gastrointestinal tract, whether slated to be converted into energy or to be eliminated as waste. Food's entry into the stomach — as well as its exit therefrom — is regulated by circular muscles which act somewhat like purse strings, alternately expanding and contracting. The stomach works on the food both mechanically and chemically. The movement of the stomach walls mashes the food, kneading it as a cook kneads dough. This permits the thorough mixing in of a digestive juice, the chief ingredients of which are pepsin and hydrochloric acid.

The stomach's principal role is that of a storage tank where food can be kept until the small intestine is ready to receive it.

Study Chart 2 a moment; notice that it shows the stomach in the center of the body although in reality the stomach lies mostly on the left side. We find the reflexes to be about even on both feet, thus we show it in the center on the chart to simplify the location of the reflexes for you. These charts are not drawn for exact accuracy of position, but more to make it convenient for the layman to find the reflexes in relation to certain parts of the body.

Now look at Fig. 12 and notice the position of the pressing of the

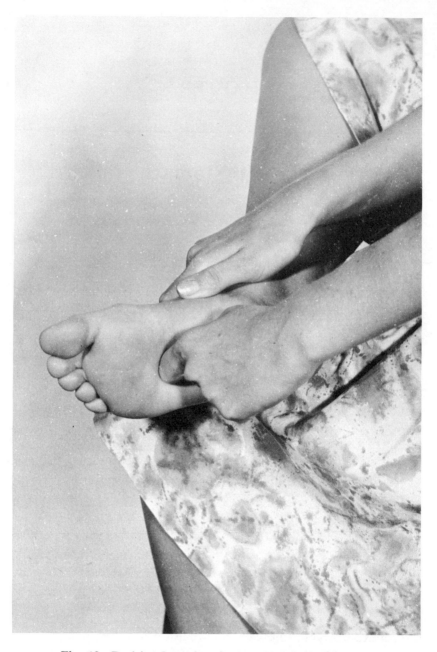

Fig. 12. Position for using the knuckle of the finger to massage the reflexes to the stomach, solar plexus, and diaphragm.

knuckle of the forefinger.

This is a handy position to use in massaging some of the reflexes. By using the knuckle you can exert more pressure in some areas, and it doesn't seem to get as tired as the thumb. If you don't have a massager or some kind of like device, then alternating the thumb and the knuckle works satisfactorily.

Let us start to massage. Since you have some idea of the workings of the stomach, you can now understand how much benefit you can give this all-important organ by stimulating it with reflex massage.

Stomach Reflex Techniques

Take the right foot up into position; bend the finger of the left hand and press the knuckle into the reflexes of the stomach as shown in Fig. 12. Press and massage with the same rolling motion that you use with the thumb. Work from the center of the foot toward the inside, clear to the spine reflexes, passing under the reflex to the thyroid. Press in and up under the pad as much as possible. Feel those tender buttons in there? You will probably find it especially tender just as you reach the spine reflex below the thyroid reflexes. This may be more sensitive because the stomach is more in the center of the body.

Does it hurt? Some of these reflexes are so tender and hurt so badly that tears will come to your eyes, or you may have to grit your teeth as you massage. But your instinct will demand that you keep on rubbing. It is Nature's call for new life, which at last you have learned how to give her, in a harmless, rejuvenating way. You can massage very gently at first, increasing the pressure as the tenderness diminishes. It will, in a surprisingly short time. Some reflexes will recover faster than others.

Remember the job your stomach has to do for you to enjoy perfect health, and the many veins and nerves running through it to keep it functioning properly.

How to Cope with Ulcers

Ulcers are very common; they afflict between 10 and 15 per cent of the population. Much mystery still surrounds them as to their origin. No one seems to know why they occur more frequently in men than in women.

Recent research has shown that some ulcers result from a malfunction of the pituitary and adrenal glands. Here we have the related action of the glands again. I hope you are beginning to understand how reflexology can bring your body back to complete health. In giving yourself these treatments, you are not only treating one malfunction that you think is causing your illness but all parts of the body, so that you are sure of getting every organ and gland back in harmony with each other.

Emotional states do not, of course, cause ulcers only, or solely afflict the digestive system. Their influence is evident in a host of ailments, ranging all the way from skin irritations, such as hives and eczema, to a fatal heart attack.

The relationship between emotions and digestion has been known for centuries: the dry mouth or empty sensation at the pit of the stomach caused by fear; the heavy stomach that accompanies depression; the cramping pain of tension. No wonder ulcers soon heal when treated with reflex massage. The whole body and mind are bathed in a soothing, relaxing sensation.

If you think you have ulcers, you will massage not only the reflexes to the stomach, but also the pituitary and adrenals to relax the emotions. Many people have recovered completely from ulcers through reflex massage.

It is said that a dog does not have ulcers, as he will go off in a dark corner and completely relax when he feels badly, and an ulcer has no power then to progress from bad to worse.

When we talk of the stomach we think of food. Do you consider your stomach when you are eating?

Reported Reflexology Healings of Ulcers

A Mr. H. had gotten his system so out of order that he actually became allergic to food of every kind. The doctors told him there was nothing they could do for him, and in desperation he turned to reflexology as a last resort. Now, several years later, he is still in perfect health.

Mr. L. was bringing a load of horses to California from New Mexico. He became very ill on the way, with bad stomach pains.

He said he had been having trouble with his stomach for the past few months but had not done anything about it. Now, he knew he would have to stop and see a doctor, but what to do with the truckload of horses? As he drove along the highway he saw a sign reading "Reflexology." He didn't know what it was but he stopped and went in. He was given a treatment; the stomach pains stopped while taking the treatment, and several years later they still had never returned.

CHAPTER 10

Reflexes to Adrenal Glands and Kidneys

Let's look at Fig. 13 for massaging the reflex to the adrenal and kidneys. In this illustration you will see the Rollo Reflex Massager being used. Notice the position and how the massager is pressed into the foot almost in the center, just above the reflex for the colon and just below the stomach and diaphragm reflexes. You have a kidney on each side of the body, so you will have a kidney and adrenal reflex on each foot.

Take the right leg and get it into position so you can easily reach the foot with the left hand. You may use the massager, your thumb, or another similar-acting device, just so you are able to press in deep enough to reach the reflex buttons under the skin. The adrenal fits on top of the kidney like a little hat, so when you massage one you will massage the other, especially if you are using one of the massagers. The kidney reflex lies lengthwise on the foot with the adrenal reflex up toward the toes. You can see that the Rollo Massager will cover larger areas of the reflexes than just the thumb or the little hand Reflex Massager. However, these may be more convenient to use when trying to find a pinpointed spot to test it for tenderness before massaging, as in the toes and the heel area.

Roll the massager (or use your hands and fingers) over the whole foot with a deep, pressing motion. When you come to a place that hurts, massage it a moment; then go on to another spot and let that spot rest. But don't forget to come back to it and give it the extra massage that it needs for another few seconds. Also, don't forget the warning about overmassaging the kidneys the first few times.

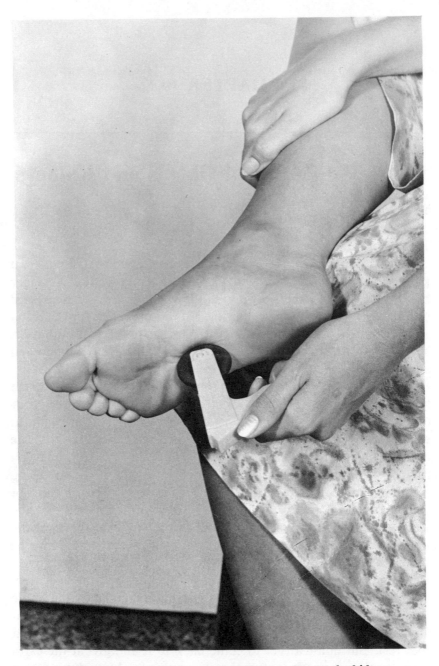

Fig. 13. Position for massaging the reflex to the kidney
and adrenal gland, using the Rollo Reflex Massager.

Be very careful of this, particularly if they are extremely tender. The kidneys are the organs which have the job of getting rid of all accumulated poison your body is throwing off as a result of this massage treatment. Treat your kidneys kindly, and give them one last little massage before you complete your treatment.

A Special Technique

The adrenal gland is one of the endocrine glands which are all related to each other. Look at Chart 3 of the endocrine glands, and keep in mind that if the reflex to any one of these glands is tender, then the others are almost sure to show some degree of tenderness also. Remember the influence the pituitary has on these other glands to keep them functioning correctly. These glands are the hormone producers, and the adrenal gland is especially influenced by a certain substance produced by the anterior lobe of the pituitary.

Many times you will find the reflex to the kidney on one foot very tender, while the reflex to the other kidney on the opposite foot will show very little or no tenderness at all. You will know definitely that the one showing the tender reflex is not contracting and relaxing as Nature intended, allowing congestion to form in that particular kidney. It does not make any difference in the reflex massage if the kidneys are overactive, causing too frequent urination, or if they are inactive, because the massaging of the reflexes to the kidneys in the center of the feet will correct and restore the kidney action to normal in a short time.

The action of the kidneys is many times influenced by fright, anger, and many kinds of distress, so it is well to give special attention to the solar plexus at this time if you feel this might be the cause of an abnormally functioning kidney. You can be the judge of this; just massage it if it hurts!

How the Kidneys Affect Various Body Parts

Also remember that the eyes may be affected by faulty kidneys. In case of eye trouble or weakness, don't forget the kidney reflexes as well as the reflexes to the eyes and neck.

Nature's tendency is to restore all normal conditions that may exist when we give her back the necessary circulation, so that she can rebuild the sick and broken-down glands and organs of the body.

While we are working on the kidney reflex, we will mention kidney stones from which it is said one out of five people suffer. In treating this condition with reflex massage, you will concentrate on relaxing the urinary tract which is the excretory duct leading from the kidney to the bladder. You can see by referring to Charts 2 and 3 approximately where the kidneys are and also the location of the bladder. Chart 2 illustrates the reflex to the bladder and Fig. 13 shows the reflex to the kidneys. Massage between these two areas, back and forth on the ureter reflex, relaxing the tension so Nature can eliminate the kidney stones through normal muscular contraction.

CHAPTER 11

Reflexes to Pancreas and Spleen

While we are learning to massage the kidney and adrenals, let us look once more at Chart 3 of the endocrine glands. Notice how the pancreas lies in between the adrenal glands. The reflex for the pancreas lies in a band extending nearly all the way across the left foot, and over halfway across the right foot, from the inside, under the big toe.

A Special Reflex Technique

To massage the reflex to the pancreas gland you will take the same position as for massaging the kidneys. You may study the chart and the illustrations; see how this gland runs across the body instead of up and down as the kidneys do. So you will massage across the foot just above the kidney reflex, about where the adrenal reflex is. You will massage more, clear across the left foot and halfway across the right foot, if you are centralizing your attention on this particular gland. But, as we have observed, the reflexes to this gland lie in about the same place that other glands lie, which are generally covered when you massage the feet in this area; hence, the gland needs little special attention. If there appears to be tenderness in any area of the pancreas, massage it out.

Many of these glands lie one behind the other in the body, so the reflexes will be confined to a small area. It is sensible not to try too hard to decide which button goes to which gland, but merely follow the rule: *When there is tenderness, massage it out.*

The pancreas gland must be treated respectfully as one of the major balancing mechanisms of your metabolism. This is the maker of insulin which lowers the sugar in the bloodstream, while adrenalin from your adrenal glands lowers it. See how interrelated they are!

Warning for Diabetics

So here is a *warning* to those who have *diabetes*. When you are using the reflex massage, you may induce a normal increase in the supply of insulin. If you are taking insulin artificially, you may have to follow the same procedure as that which would be used for insulin shock, for which your physician would recommend an immediate intake of additional sugar. This has happened many times when I gave people treatments. In some cases they did not tell me of the diabetes until later.

There are so many people who do not know that they have diabetes and only live half a life. Many times grief or shock will so affect the entire glandular system that the result will be diabetes. This type of diabetes will usually respond to reflex massage and not take as many treatments as a long-standing case of diabetes will require.

Diabetes in children is sometimes caused by something that happened to the mother before they were born. Doctors tell us there is no cure for these children. However, we know that reflex massage cannot hurt, it only benefits Nature in her attempt to heal the body by giving her a normal circulatory system. I would say have faith and massage anyway. I have seen some marvelous things happen that surprised me many times when doctors had said it couldn't be done.

Don't forget to look for tenderness in other gland reflexes, especially the thyroid glands and the pituitary.

Reflex for the Spleen

Next we will take a look at the spleen in Chart 2. See how it is located on the left side, touching the left kidney close to the spine.

It will be seen on the chart that the reflex button to the spleen is in about the same position on the left foot as the gallbladder reflex button is on the right foot, except that it is slightly closer to the outer edge of the foot. Look at the illustration, "Reflexes for the Heart" (Fig. 15, page 78); use this position, holding the left foot and massaging with the right hand. This will be a smaller area to massage than for the pancreas reflex. Since it lies under the reflex for the heart, it will generally get its share of massage when you are massaging the heart reflex.

Anemic Conditions

If you find that the reflex area for the spleen has any tenderness at all, then you are probably somewhat anemic. Anyone who is anemic will find a tenderness in this region with no difficulty. Improvement can be so rapid it is amazing. With pernicious anemia, results will be slower, but Nature will be there, changing new blood cells for old.

The spleen serves as a storehouse for iron needed by the blood. The intestinal peristalsis is powerfully stimulated by a substance produced by the spleen which acts upon both the large and small intestines. The spleen is believed to absorb the particles of broken-down red corpuscles, and is a storehouse for additional iron needed by the blood.

Cause of Anemia

Anemia is caused by lack of iron in the blood and can cause serious trouble if neglected for a long period of time. Women are more prone to be anemic than men. When I was very young I became very anemic but didn't have any idea what my trouble was. I just didn't seem to have the energy to climb out of bed, let alone walk around. The doctor said that because I was so anemic I had the energy of an 80-year-old woman. Do you ever feel like that? Massage the spleen reflex to see if you can find tenderness. If there is, then you have congestion and the spleen is not working properly. So massage it out.

One day while walking down the street, I started having pains below the little toe near the heart reflex. The pains kept bothering me, so I stooped down as if to fix my shoe, slipped my shoe off, and gave the spot a few quick digs with my finger. The pains stopped. When I got home, I sat down, picked up my left foot, and pressed around to make sure of where the warning pains had come from. I found the spot very quickly on the reflex to the spleen. Then I realized that I must have become anemic, so I massaged the area thoroughly until most of the tenderness was gone. A little later I accidentally cut my finger and I could see that my blood was not the rich, dark red that it should have been. Thus warned, I concentrated on iron-rich food, iron tonic, and massage of the reflex to the spleen. Physically, I never knew that I had been anemic.

CHAPTER 12

How to Handle Reflexes for the Liver

By now you have learned the correct techniques for contacting the various reflex buttons in the feet as far as we have gone. We have been working on the reflexes which have included both feet; now we come to the liver, which is located only on the right foot as you will see by looking at Chart 2.

Take your right foot and get it into position for massaging. Notice in Fig. 14, "Reflexes to the liver," how the thumb of the left hand is pressing on the pad just under the little toe. This is the area of the liver reflexes. Massage this area with a rolling, pressing motion. It could be said that the liver reflex consists of several buttons to contact, for this is a large gland to cover with reflexes.

The liver is the largest gland in the body. It weighs about 3 pounds in an adult, and has within it at all times about one-quarter of all the blood in the body, circulating through it.

The liver performs many tasks, such as being a great filter; it is a natural antiseptic and purgative; it manufactures bile to digest fats and prevent constipation, forming about 2 pints of bile a day. This goes into the intestines to lubricate and prevent constipation. It also helps to supply some of the substances for blood making, and stores up sugar within itself for future uses.

If you find tenderness in this area, indicating a sluggish liver, it will be more in the nature of a dull pain, rather than the sharp pains characterizing other reflexes you have previously massaged. You will then know that the liver is sluggish and lacks the proper circulation and muscular action to function properly. When the

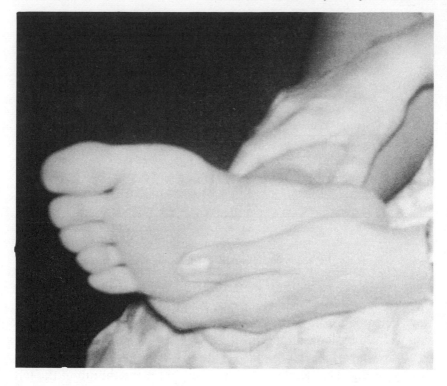

Fig. 14. Position for massaging the reflexes to the liver.

normal function of this important gland has been neglected over a long period of time it can result in diabetes, gallstones, jaundice, atrophy, sclerosis, constipation, etc. There is no doubt of the wonderful healing results you can obtain by massaging the reflex to the liver. So continue massaging with a firm, rolling pressure, so that the natural circulation can be restored by dissolving the accumulated crystals, lessening the obstruction to good health.

Warning About a Sluggish Liver

Let me warn you about a very sluggish liver, which would be very sensitive to the touch. Massage it very lightly, and for only a second the first time. You can expect several different reactions from this treatment for the liver. In severe cases it is best not to massage the reflexes of the liver again for several days, giving Nature a chance to throw off excess poison and adjust itself to increased circulation which you have put in motion by massaging these reflexes.

Some people have felt very relieved after the first treatment, and then when they took the second massage of the liver reflexes, became quite ill as Nature goes to work to eliminate the excess poison released by the congested liver. After the third treatment taken three days later, they always feel much better and show a lot of improvement with each treatment thereafter.

I have had patients have 10 and 12 bowel movements in one day after the second or third treatment. The stools at this time may be of heavy mucus, black, green, or other off colors. This is Nature doing her long-delayed house cleaning. During this time you may have a tired, listless feeling. Don't worry, think how well you will feel when Nature has completed her cleaning job.

Massage this pad under the little toe on the right foot and feel for any tenderness in the area. If the liver is enlarged, we will find a larger area of the foot involved. Remember our motto, "If it hurts, massage it."

How to Cope with Gallbladder Conditions

While you have the right foot in this position, let's massage the reflexes to the gallbladder. Notice on Chart 2 how the gallbladder is just a little below and toward the center of the liver reflex. This gallbladder is lodged on the undersurface of the right lobe of the liver, and is a pear-shaped, fibro-muscular receptacle for the bile. This is also the receptacle where the very painful, hardened masses called gallstones are found. There are many cases where reflex massage of the liver and gallbladder have saved people from having an operation, with the stones seeming to vanish after a few treatments. It is not known whether these stones have dissolved or whether the treatments so relax the gall duct that they are passed off.

If you find any tenderness in this area at all, massage it with either the thumb or hand massager, until every bit of tenderness is gone. Don't try to rub it all out the first time, though. It took a long time to get congested, so give Nature her chance to relieve this congestion, which you will know has taken place when the tenderness is no longer there.

Case History of Chronic Fatigue Overcome

Mr. S. was a great, big, handsome man over 6 feet tall, with a large frame. His wife was about 4 feet, 6 inches tall and had worked hard all her life supporting him and the children. He had always been too sick to work, I was told by his relatives who had recommended him to me. Just plain lazy was the only disease that Jim had, they said in disgust. I could see why they felt this way by looking at the two.

No person is just plain lazy, I told them. Everyone wants to feel full of vitality. No one is happy just lying around; it is against Nature. We were born to use our bodies, to work and play and find joy in living. A so-called "lazy" person is really sick. Somewhere in his body there is congestion of glands or organs that is cutting off a healthy circulation of the very life forces that keep us alive. Never condemn a lazy person; he is to be pitied.

Lazy people lie around without any show of energy and they certainly are not filled with a zest for life. They don't want to work, but they don't play either. Their life is very empty. They don't know why they are this way. They are condemned about it on every side, as if they are that way on purpose. And they readily agree that they are lazy, just as heavy people will agree that they are overweight. *Lazy* should have another synonym denoting loss of energy as other health problems have. Reflexology can help reclaim their true energy.

Mr. S. came to me for treatments for several weeks and didn't show the improvement that I thought he should. He did have several glands that were not functioning properly according to my findings in the reflexes of his feet, thus the feet were very tender in some places. But Mr. S. was a baby where pain was concerned. He wiggled and twisted and moaned every time that I barely touched a tender spot any place on his feet. So I did massage very gently. In fact, I didn't feel that I was doing him much good, because I could not break up the crystals in the capillaries so that they could free the bloodstream of the congestion or stopped-up lines that were slowing a free flow of healing blood to depleted glands and organs. And also, I could not exert enough pressure to send the electrical life force surging through his body to recharge his vitality enough to build up his energy.

One day after I had him seated in the chair with his shoes and socks removed, I said, "Jim, you are not improving as you should, and it is because I have been too easy on you. Today I am going to give you a good working over and get something stirred up in there. Can you take it?" He said he could.

I dug in, starting with the pituitary reflex in the center of his big toe. That had improved considerably during the time he had been coming, even though I had not massaged it very heavily. The thyroid had improved somewhat, too. As I went over each reflex I massaged quite deeply, and he sat there and hung onto the chair arms gritting his teeth but taking it like a man. Then I came to the liver reflex, my fingers pressing into the spongy area under the little toe on the right side. I thought I had lost both arms of my chair for sure. A congested, sluggish liver. What could make a person more tired than a malfunctioning liver? No wonder the poor man was called lazy all of his life. He wasn't lazy; he was sick, not enough to be sick in bed or complain about it, but he had a reason for his chronic fatigue.

Of course, the adrenals and the thyroid had a place in this lack of energy, too. And also, since the whole mechanism of the body was out of balance for probably most of his existence because of the glands that did not function as they should, Mr. S. had not lived a very pleasant life. I don't suppose he enjoyed seeing his little wife get out and support him and the children for most of their married years. But if you are so tired that it is an effort to stoop down to pick up the paper, is it fair for us more fortunate people to call others lazy?

From then on, Mr. S. improved very rapidly and the tender spots in the bottoms of his feet vanished almost completely.

So remember to look to the reflexes of the liver to alleviate any feeling of chronic sluggishness and lack of energy. Check the adrenals and thyroid also for any sign of tenderness.

CHAPTER 13

Conditioning Reflexes for the Heart

There probably would be no argument over the fact that the heart is one of the more important organs in the body. Here is the pump which must send blood to the remotest parts of the body. The heart is a strong muscle, made to endure with ease and efficiency.

You will see as you study Charts 1 and 2 that the heart is located on the left side of the body, a part of it even extending over into the center. Remember this when you are massaging the heart reflexes.

Lift your left leg up so that you can easily reach the left foot with the right hand. (See Fig. 15 for locating reflex to the heart.)

Notice how the thumb is pressed into the pad under the little toe, just as you did on the right foot for the liver reflex. Press and massage this whole area, searching for tender spots. When you find any part that is tender, then massage it out, covering the area thoroughly — for, *if congestion in any degree is allowed to remain in the arteries and veins surrounding the heart for a long enough period, the result might be a heart attack.*

Relaxation with Reflexology

No matter what the nature of the trouble is, the heart can be aided with the reflex push buttons. The results relax all muscles and veins. How often I have treated heart complaints with reflex massage while we waited for the doctor to arrive, or until I was

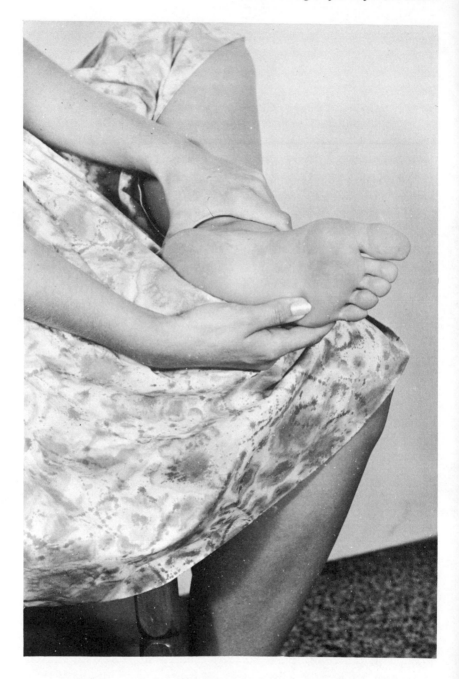

Fig. 15. Position for massaging the reflex to the heart.

satisfied the afflicted one was out of danger and free from discomfort.

My reflexology instructor asked during class one day if any of her students, in the course of working on a person suffering from heart trouble, had noticed that person cry out when a sharp pain went from foot to heart, followed by the sensation of a stimulant. It was surprising to see some ten or more students signify that they had.

Further investigation revealed that some cases showed the heart patient was never again troubled, even when his difficulties had been severe. If there is pain around the heart, or in the chest region, the entire area of reflexes should be worked on. If the condition seems to be angina pectoris, characterized by pains going up the arm and shoulder, work clear to the base of the little toe and on top of it, as you would for the shoulder. Also work up to the root of the fourth and fifth toes.

It should not take long to find the exact button which is crying for pressing and massaging, to release the congestion.

Some Causes of Death from Heart Trouble

Probably too often death is declared to be from heart failure when actually it was the poor condition of other glands which caused the heart to give out from overwork.

People fill their bodies with unfit foods. They put an extra load on the heart by filling the lungs with nicotine. The list would be long if one were to jot down all the small items of daily living which tax the heart until it gives up. It is truly said that death overtakes one in "small bites."

This marvelous pumping station is located between the lungs and is enclosed in the cavity of the pericardium. It is embedded deep in the body. Often the reflex buttons will take more pressure than in other cases because of this. The heart covers quite an area in the upper portion of the chest cavity, to the left, and so it is that there will be several reflex buttons, corresponding with the different parts of the heart or around it.

If you are troubled with a heart condition, you will find it simpler to use the Reflex Massager, as it does the work of massaging the reflexes with ease and puts no strain on you. Yes, it may be possible to massage one's heartaches away!

Cases of Recoveries from Heart Trouble

I can give you many case histories of wonderful results from this scientific massage of the reflexes on heart patients. But this is one that I am going to give you as a warning. *Don't overdo! Never overdo!*

A Mr. B. came to me for treatments for a heart condition that he had suffered for quite a while. With all his medicines, he was in and out of bed, and very weak from being inactive for so long. Remember that the heart is a muscle and when your outer muscles become flabby, so do the inner muscles, too, like the heart. If your legs and arms were very soft from lying around for several months, you wouldn't try to go out and play several games of tennis, ball, or golf, just because you felt good one day, would you? If you did, you would probably have muscle spasms in your arms and legs all night.

Now, the heart is a muscle, too, a big muscle. Twenty-four quarts of blood pass through the circulatory system in three minutes. In a male, the heart weighs from 10 to 12 ounces in proportion to the size of the body. If you overtaxed it with unusual exercise before giving it a chance to build up strength after a long rest, it could very easily have a muscle spasm, too — heart attack! This often happens when retired men go on hunting trips, etc.

Mr. B. took about three treatments from me in a period of seven days. He felt so well that he decided he would go to work. He was sure he was well, which he very surely could have been, but his heart was still very soft from months of inactivity. I told him repeatedly, "Wait a while, give yourself time to get strong, don't rush it. Give your heart a chance." That same week he went to the factory to ask for his old job back. He drove the car over 100 miles. He felt like a new man, he said. He walked all over the big factory, up many flights of stairs and down again.

His old boss was glad to have him back and was showing him around. On the way back to the car he had to walk up a long hill, and then is when his heart began to protest. After that he was back to his old up and down routine. He never came back to me. He lost faith in this great work that might have made him a healthy man the rest of his life. If he had only listened to my warning, or even used common sense.

Don't you be a Mr. B, no matter how well you get to feeling after massaging your reflexes. Take a little time, give your body a chance to build up strength and muscle, and you will be able to stay a "new man" all of your life.

Case History of Heart and Stress Conditions Eased

Mr. H. came to me with several complaints, the most pressing one being a heart condition caused by rheumatic fever which he had suffered when he was a child, in addition to a nervous stomach. He had spent much of his time in hospitals and had been bedfast for months at a time. He was married, with several children to support, and this affliction made life very hard on him and his family. Luckily he owned his own business, but it suffered setbacks when he had attacks and would have to remain in bed for several weeks at a time. This caused him to go into a mental depression which in addition to his heart condition caused a vicious circle of disharmony in the body.

His nerves were in a terrible condition and he was plainly under strong mental stress. In fact, he had become so bad that he would have crying spells for no reason. He could not relax enough to fall asleep at night, which added to his condition because we all know that the body heals while we sleep. He had no appetite, showing a depression of digestive activities. He suffered from constipation. In plain words, he was a physical wreck and the only future he had to look forward to was to get worse and to finally end up in an early grave. Mr. H. was only in his early 30's at the time he came to me for treatments, as mentioned before, to see if I could bring him some relief for his stomach, as eating had become a serious problem for him.

You have probably known people like this that seem to go from bad to worse, at last hopelessly giving up their life. Mr. H. proceeded to tell me of all his ailments and complaints as I started to massage his very tender feet. He wouldn't have had to tell me his problems because they were all there in the bottoms of his feet. I felt that they were screaming for help as I massaged each reflex very gently. With a warm feeling of pleasure, I watched this poor, distressed man quiet down as I worked on the reflexes, especially those to the endocrine glands. Remember, I had to be very careful not to overmassage any particular reflex area the first time due to his bad condition, so I spent a few minutes just massaging the whole foot with my open hand while I watched him drop off to sleep for a few minutes.

It was a pleasure to watch Mr. H. regaining his health, as the stimulation of massaging the reflexes started his congested glands and organs back to normal functioning. I renewed the circulation in his whole body by massaging all of the reflexes in both feet. Thus not just one of his many symptoms began to show improvement, but we were rewarded by his overall return to health. When he came to me the first time he had been despondent and without hope. The first thing that his wife noticed was his renewed sense of well being. Almost at once his disposition improved and she told me later that instead of crying, he was cheerful and better natured than she had seen him since their early marriage. And she said he would fall asleep as soon as his head hit the pillow, something that he had not been able to do for years.

All of this added up to an increase of vitality in the whole mechanism of his body. His stomach improved rapidly and he was able to eat again without discomfort as soon as the disturbances of the digestive tract had been helped back to a normal functioning when stimulated by the reflexes.

As his glands began to respond to the stimulation, Mr. H's whole body took on new life. He found that he was no longer constipated and could give up taking harsh laxatives. And as each organ and gland relaxed, it freed the mind from a nervous tension condition as the system recuperated, taking the load of tension off the straining heart.

Doctors had always warned him that he could not do the things other men did. He must remain a semi-invalid all of his life if he wanted to live at all. His heart returned to normal enough to allow him to do anything that he wanted to do without any trouble from it. His blood pressure returned to normal; his eyes sparkled with health and the joy of being healthy for the first time since he was a small boy.

Today, after more than ten years have passed, he is a strong and well man, running a large, successful business, besides enjoying sports in his spare time, such as fishing and hunting, etc.

What did I do to make a new man of Mr. H? Well, the first thing that I worked on was the reflex to the pituitary gland which is in the center of the big toe if you remember your chart. This is the main gland of the whole body — the king gland.

Then I dropped on down to the reflex of the thyroid which is just below the big toe; then I massaged the thymus in the center of the foot for a second; then on down the foot to the adrenal reflexes; from there to the gonads or sex glands under the ankles; then my fingers searched out the reflexes to the spleen, which is the storehouse of energy and the red blood builder. I went from one foot to the other, making sure I only pressed on each reflex two or three times at the most.

I stimulated the endocrine glands first. Then I carefully worked on the rest of the reflexes, such as heart, liver, kidneys, and the eyes and ear area and the sinus reflexes, as he was also afflicted with a bad case of sinus trouble. The whole body was out of harmony, out of tune, and we merely helped Nature put it back in tune by massaging the reflexes and giving her a chance to bring new life to all of the congested glands and dying cells in the body. Thus health was quickly and simply restored through reflexology.

CHAPTER 14

Solar Plexus Reflexes

The solar plexus is situated behind the stomach and in front of the diaphragm. So when we massage the stomach reflexes we are bound to also massage these two reflexes, although they will be reached more in the center of the feet, as the solar plexus is located in the center of the body.

This great network of nerves goes out to all parts of the abdominal cavity, and is sometimes called the abdominal brain. The fine network of nerves extends from the part of the aorta below the diaphragm, and includes the front of the abdominal aorta, as well as the adrenal glands.

Special Techniques

To massage this reflex to the solar plexus you will take the same position as for the stomach reflex massage. Notice in the illustration for stomach reflexes (Fig. 12, page 58), the location of the finger on the foot. It is not quite centered, so move the finger over toward the middle of the foot. You may find it easier to use the thumb for this relaxing position. Instead of the rolling motion, here we are going to use a slow push-and-release motion.

Get the right foot into position. Now place the thumb of your left hand on the solar plexus reflex. Push in gradually while taking a breath slowly into your lungs as you press the solar plexus button; hold for a second; then use a slow releasing motion, as you slowly release your breath at the same time. Do this a few times; then change to the left foot and repeat. You will feel such a rewarding sense of relaxation that you may fall asleep. It might be good to use this as one of your last massages so you can lie down for a nap or rest. If you have someone to help you, it is good to do this massage on both feet at the same time.

Massaging the Diaphragm Reflex

It is impossible to massage the reflex to the solar plexus without affecting the one to the diaphragm, which is a muscular wall acting as a partition to separate the thorax from the abdomen.

Every time a muscle contracts, it has a squeezing effect on the blood vessels, especially the veins. It will be obvious how the circulatory system is benefited. So when you massage this particular area, you are sending aid to the important nerve centers of the body.

CHAPTER 15

Reflexing the Appendix and Ileocecal Valve

It could be safely stated that the appendix is one of the best-known organs, although it is a tube no more than 3 to 6 inches long lying below the waist and on the right side.

Proper Reflex Techniques

To massage the reflex to the appendix, let's take a look at the picture for massage of reflexes to the appendix and ileocecal valve in Fig. 16. Notice how the thumb is pressed in about halfway along the foot from heel to toes, and quite close to the outer edge of the foot. To locate the reflex to this wormlike organ, you will have to do a little exploring. If there is no congestion in the appendix or inflammation in the ileocecal valve, then you will not be able to find it, but don't worry as they are so centrally located that they will get enough massage to keep them in good, healthy condition.

To massage the appendix reflexes, which you know will be on the right foot as the appendix is on the right side of the body, lift the right foot into position as shown in Fig. 16. Now press in the area shown in the picture with a rolling motion, until you hit the button under the skin that will give you the pain signal that there is trouble here. You will probably have to move your thumb, or massaging device, around a bit on this particular reflex before you find it.

It seems to be in a little different area on different people, but not over a quarter of an inch one way or the other. When you do

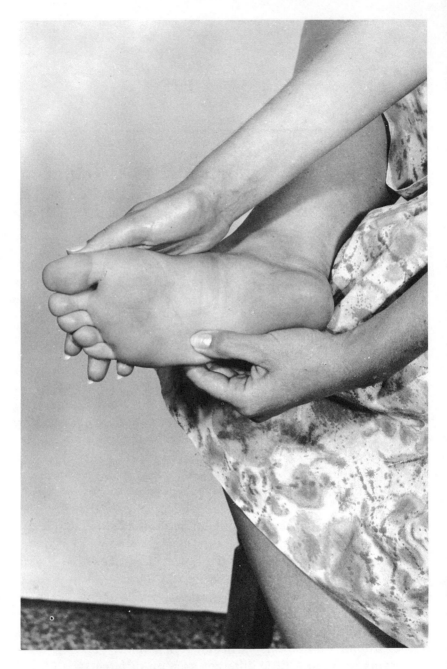

Fig. 16. Position for massaging the reflexes to the appendix and ileocecal valve.

find it, massage for a few seconds; then let it rest while you massage some other area, then come back to it and massage a few more seconds. Do this each time you massage your reflexes until all tenderness has vanished.

Reported Recoveries from Appendicitis

Many marvelous recoveries from appendicitis have been experienced because of the massaging of the reflexes for this organ. In case of an acute attack, the attention of a physician would be needed, of course. But you may massage the appendix reflex until he arrives, as it will relax the inflamed area involved.

A friend of mine did not believe in this reflex system of healing, although she sent many of her friends to me for treatments. One day I went to visit her and found her lying on her bed in much pain. "I've got appendicitis," she moaned, "call the doctor!" I said, "I will not call the doctor until you let me see your feet. I don't believe you have appendicitis at all." I went over and picked up her right foot, pressed on the reflex to the appendix, and found there was no tenderness. Then I moved on up to the reflex to the stomach and solar plexus and found this area somewhat tender. I massaged it for just a few seconds, she expelled some gas, and the pain was completely gone. She couldn't believe it; she kept marveling at how it could go so suddenly.

Always after that visit, when I went to see her she would kick off her shoes so I could give her feet a reflex massage.

The Important Ileocecal Valve

Tenderness in this particular region of the foot, however, can sometimes indicate trouble other than in the appendix. The ileocecal valve forms the opening from the small intestine into the colon. This opening is toward the large intestine and guards against reflex from the large into the small bowel. This is an important little portion, especially if you are inclined to suffer from an allergy.

A Case of Food Allergy Healed

Mr. C. had been a seaman all his life and enjoyed his type of work, but through the years he had developed an allergy to various foods served at sea. At first he did not pay much attention to the distress, but as time passed he became increasingly worse until it seemed that everything he ate made him break out with hives or gave him indigestion. Finally he had to give up his life on the seas — he had reached the point where he was afraid to eat anything. Doctors had given him tests, and he had been taking shots and pills until he said he had become allergic even to them. He had tried everything else, he told me, and wanted to see if reflexology was the answer.

When I took his feet in my hands, I found all of the reflexes extremely tender. After carefully massaging the endocrine reflexes for a few seconds, I moved my fingers to the spot under the second toe (from the big toe). This was so tender that he could barely stand to have me touch it, but using my "feather touch" I worked on all the toes, one by one, rolling and twisting them gently between my fingers.

Then I concentrated on the *ileocecal valve* reflex. This is located in the same position as the appendix reflex, and he moaned out loud with pain as my fingers barely pressed the spot. Notice in Chart 2 how it is situated slightly toward the outer edge from the center of the foot.

When Mr. C. got home, he called me to tell me that he felt much better already and that he felt he was really going to recover his health.

When he came back in two days, he looked so much better that I was amazed at the change. He had lost his gray pallor, and his face was no longer drawn and haggard. He said he had slept soundly for the past two nights, and though he was still wary about food, his meals had caused him little distress.

It was surprising to see how few treatments it took to put Mr. C. back on the road to living a healthy, normal life once more. He insists that reflexology saved his very life. Now, several years later, he is completely free of all food allergies, eats whatever he wants to, and enjoys perfect health, all thanks to Nature's own simple way of restoring the organs and glands to normalcy.

Case History of a Sinus Condition Healed

A Mr. M. came to me with a bad case of sinus. His head had become so stuffed up that he was unable to go to work for days at a time. Since he was a businessman and had to face the public, it made it very embarrassing for him to face them when he could not close his mouth, but had to keep it open in order to breathe.

Of course, he had all of the other symptoms that go with sinuses, such as headaches, poor hearing at times, nervousness and irritability, upset stomach, etc. Naturally the reflexes indicated all of this the first time I gave him a treatment.

After I had gone over both of his feet and massaged each and every tender reflex, I concentrated on the ileocecal valve reflex located in the same area that we find the reflex to the appendix, on the right foot a little up toward the toes from the center of the foot and just a little toward the outside of the foot. If you are troubled with sinus of any kind you will have no trouble in locating this reflex, as it will shock you with pain when it is pressed firmly with the thumb or a like device so as to press in deeply enough to reach the button under the skin.

Next I massaged all of the reflexes under the toes, which were extremely sore, especially the reflex just at the bottom of the second toe from the big toe. See Fig. 9 (page 39) and also Chart 1 for this position, as it seems to be the main one that will loosen the congestion of sinus in the head, and it doesn't seem to matter how long this particular reflex is massaged if you are careful not to bruise the capillaries (tiny blood vessels) in the skin.

I noticed Mr. M. seemed to be getting relief on the left side of his head as I massaged the reflexes in the left foot. Suddenly he could breathe through his nostril on the left side. "Boy, what a relief," he exclaimed.

Then I went to work on the right foot and massaged the reflexes under the toes again as I had done on the left foot. After some time of massaging, the right side of his head opened up so that he was able to also breathe through the right nostril. He was so elated and surprised at the results, he said, "I didn't really believe this would help when I came in here." He told me, "I almost changed my mind and canceled the appointment, it seemed so ridiculous."

I laughingly told him that I heard those same words every day, but the sad thing was some people actually did back out at the last minute from lack of faith in the method of reflex massage, and that it always made me feel badly for this person who had come so close to such a simple and natural way back to health and then missed it.

After I had helped Mr. M. breathe normally again, I asked him about his back. I had noticed that it was extremely tender in one area, as I had been covering his reflexes in the general massage.

He told me that he had a slipped disc according to the doctors and that it was getting worse fast. The doctors had told him that nothing but an operation could help him, and that it was a very serious and dangerous operation. He said that he knew he was going to have to give up and have it done soon, but dreaded it. "Too bad these treatments aren't magic enough to fix my back, too," he said jokingly.

"What makes you think they can't?" I asked him. "You didn't believe that they could help your sinuses an hour ago, and look at you now! Why couldn't they do as much for your back or any other part of your body for that matter?"

He looked at me in real surprise. "You mean they really could?" he asked in amazement. "Don't you think that they could?" I asked him seriously. "Yes, I do believe they can if you say so; after opening up my head like they have, I would believe that they could do anything. I will come back every day for a treatment," he said. I had to explain to him that one treatment every other day was all that he should take for the first week anyway, so he was content to come back in two days.

Mr. M. came faithfully for his treatments every week after his first week of taking one every other day. Sometimes his wife would call me at seven o'clock in the morning and ask if I would give Mr. M. a treatment for his sinus condition so he could go to work that day, when he would have an attack in between treatments. His allergies did not vanish in a week. His body had taken a long time to get into that state, and it took a little while to put it back into a condition that was once more in tune with the universe.

Remember this truth if your health does not become perfect as soon as you want it to. It has been neglected for a long time by forgetting Nature's reflexes as the way to keep the circulation flowing freely so as to loosen and banish all congestion from the body.

When Mr. M. came over for special massage on the sinus reflexes, I concentrated on the toes. Sometimes I would massage the reflex at the base of the second and third toes for over an hour before we could break the congestion loose, but when we finally succeeded he was able to go to work free from any signs of congestion in his head, which might not bother him again for some time.

As we kept up the massage of the reflexes, he noticed a great improvement in his back also. Within a year he was able to take long hikes up and down mountains, carrying large, heavy objects. He was able to paint his home, climbing ladders and carrying paint, etc. And in two years he roofed his house, carrying heavy bundles of roofing up high ladders, with no recurrences of the back trouble he had complained of before he had the reflex massage treatments.

Don't underestimate the power of reflex massage, no matter what your complaint. It cannot hurt to try it and your reward will probably be a satisfactory recovery.

CHAPTER 16

Reflexes to the Small Intestine

This chapter is concerned with learning a little about the small intestine. Notice in Chart 2 at the beginning of this book how the small intestine seems to fill the lower abdomen. This intestine is the longest of the gastrointestinal tract, a channel so coiled and twisted upon itself that it winds and bends for more than 20 feet. You will note that the reflexes to the small intestine are located in the heel, and because they cover such a large area it is wise to massage the whole pad of the heel. You will note in Chart 2 how the colon makes almost a complete circle around the small intestine. Keep this in mind when massaging the reflexes to the small intestine. The reflexes are found from the heel line almost up to the waistline, and all the way across from the inside almost to the outside of the foot.

Special Reflex Techniques

You are to massage each foot in this area. If the Reflex Massager is used, it would be better to use the blunt side to cover the whole area more completely. If you find pinpoints of tenderness, then massage the buttons under the skin with the blunt tip of the hand Reflex Massager, or you may use the sharp tip if it seems hard to reach. This is where the Rollo Massager helps in your massage, too; but you can cover the area with the thumb or the knuckle of the finger if you have nothing else to work with and feel that there is congestion in the small intestine.

95

Take one foot up in position and start your deep, rolling motion at the heel, working back and forth across the foot until you get up to the waistline of the foot. As the heel has a heavier layer of skin in most cases, you will probably have to use the knuckle or some equally hard device to press in deeply enough to do any good.

The food that you have swallowed and taken into the stomach passes on into this 20 feet of intestine. That is a long length of intestine tissue to become congested, so hasten the healing process by massaging the reflexes. You will be amazed how quickly you will get relief from gastric disturbances, flatulence, etc.

CHAPTER 17

Reflexes to the Colon

Now we come to the colon, in tracing the intestinal system. The small intestine at last deposits the waste of our food into the large intestine or colon, where it is forced through the rectum, and by a series of final contractions is forced from the body as wastes.

The colon is about twice the diameter of the small intestine. The site of the first part of the colon is best known because the appendix opens into it close to the junction with the small intestine and the ileocecal valve. We have already seen on Chart 2 how the wormlike appendix is attached and how the colon stretches upward from the right lower corner of the abdomen. From there it curves just below the liver to course across the upper abdomen as the transverse colon, descending on the left side to vend into the coils of what is called the sigmoid flexure, and from there joining the rectum.

How the Colon Works

Bacteria are numerous in the colon. Their presence is important to the body because of their ability to build up such essential substances as vitamin K, needed for blood coagulation, and several components of vitamin B. At times the continuous taking of antibacterial drugs, which sterilize the intestine, has resulted in vitamin K deficiency.

The colon is the final canal for the food to travel through. What remains of the food solution spends 10 to 12 hours in the large intestine, losing large quantities of water. As a final step, the solution is attacked by a colony of bacteria to decay the remains of what started out as a meal.

This is the garbage pail of the body, and should be emptied at least once or twice a day. Animals empty their colon many times a day. The colon is truly the seat of many illnesses. Keep it emptied and clean for good health.

Colon Reflex Techniques

Let us start massaging the colon by lifting the right foot up into position, since the colon has its beginning at the end of the small intestine low down on the right side of the abdomen. With the thumb of the right hand, instead of the left, you will press near the outside of the foot just above the pad of the heel and work up toward the waistline of the foot with your pressing, rolling motion.

I suggest that you use the thumb or finger of the right hand for this position, as it seems to give you more power than you would have with the left hand which we use in other positions. You will soon learn which position is the most convenient for you — use it. If you have one of the massagers, it will simplify most of your massaging greatly.

You should now be at the "waistline" of the foot, still using your pressing, rolling motion to go across the foot toward the center and work to the reflexes of the spine. Work this area several times, hunting for buttons that will give you pain signals telling you something is wrong. When you do find these tender spots, massage them a few seconds each. Keep in mind that pain suggests congestion, and by massaging that particular reflex it will release a supply of life-giving blood, hastening the healing process, thus relieving the congested tissues.

Now we have the remainder of the colon on the left side of the body, as you will see on Chart 2. Lift the left leg up into position. We will use the right hand for massage again on this foot. It will be best to start at the waistline of the foot on the inside next to the reflexes of the spine and work toward the outer edge of the foot, as we follow the colon in its natural travel across the foot toward the descending colon.

You may find some spots along here that will make you wince with pain at the slightest pressure. Massage them gently at first, increasing the pressure as the pain subsides. Continue the same rolling, massaging motion on down the outside of the left foot, following the course of the descending colon in the body on down to the pad of the heel. You cannot be sure that it is the colon or some other organ that is sending out the pain messages as you massage over certain areas. Don't let this concern you; just keep in mind, where congestion exists, disease will result. Massage it out.

As the world-famous surgeon, the late Sir W.A. Lane said: "There is but one disease, insufficient drainage — inadequate elimination of poisonous waste material. Unless it is thrown off, poisonous waste remains in the system and begins slowly to undermine the health of our organism, finally destroying it." Is this happening to you? Now you know what to do about it.

Varicose Veins

Varicose veins are also helped through the massage of the colon and the liver reflexes. I have brought lasting relief to sufferers of varicose veins by starting the proper circulation with reflex massage, thus causing the congestion to disappear. This is true also with cramps or pains of any kind in the legs.

CHAPTER 18

Reflex to the Bladder

The bladder is a closed sac into whose lower neckline portion the ureters empty. The ureters are two hollow, thin-walled tubes about the caliber of a pencil. They connect the kidneys to the bladder, one tube coming from each kidney into the bladder. Urine cannot run down the ureter by gravity, since passage through it must continue even when we are lying down. Urine is moved along by peristalsis, waves of contracting circular muscle similar to those that expel material from the bronchi or the intestine.

The bladder whose function it is to store urine for periodic release, changes position and shape according to the amount of filling. When it is empty, the bladder is flat or concave on top and inclines forward. When it is full, it becomes rounded and projects upward. It is composed of a smooth muscle coat like that of the intestine, but of greater thickness. The urethra is the tubelike passage which conducts the urine from the bladder to the exterior and expels the urine.

Techniques for Bladder Reflex

Study Chart 2 and notice how the bladder lies in the lower lumbar region. The reflexes to the bladder will be in the same place as the reflexes to the rectum and end of the spine, only not so deep. Notice the illustration of reflexes to the bladder in Fig. 17.

The thumb is pressed into the soft, hollow part on the inside of the foot, almost next to the pad of the heel. You will be able to feel a soft, spongy area about as large as a quarter. The thumb is positioned so as to massage the bladder, and with a rolling motion, massage on up the ureter tube to the kidney. Massage this a few times also.

Lift either foot up into position for massaging, as the reflex to the bladder will be on both feet in the same location, since the bladder is located in the center of the body. Now, you have the foot ready to be massaged. You will notice in the picture that we again use the hand on the same side as the foot we are massaging — right foot, right hand; left foot, left hand. The thumb will press into the bladder reflex almost naturally. Massage with a gentle, circular motion any part that is tender.

If you are having trouble with the bladder and do not seem to find a tender spot in this area, keep massaging and pressing a little deeper until you do touch the reflex button, which will give you a pain signal that you are on the right spot. This reflex is so near the location of the rectum, prostate, and lower spine reflexes that you will not be able to tell the difference except for depth in massaging. For these reflexes you will probably have to use the Reflex Hand Massager or like device in order to press hard enough to reach these particular buttons. It's just like reaching through the front of your pelvis to reach the end of the spine or rectum.

Bladder Disorders Helped

Massage the whole spongy area for the bladder reflex on the surface. Cystitis (inflammation of the bladder) will work out very quickly and usually you will notice a great improvement after the first treatment. All sensation of burning and itching usually disappears completely after the second or third treatment. Any sensation of irritation in the bladder area will be benefited by massaging these reflexes. Remember, if at any time in any area there is bleeding, and it persists after the third treatment or after a week of treatments, consult your physician to make sure there is no malignancy present.

I have had so many wonderful results from massaging the reflexes to the bladder, by relaxing tension and breaking up

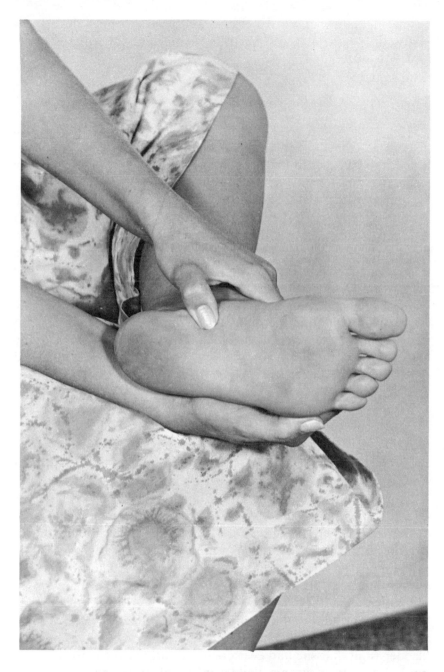

Fig. 17. Position for massaging the reflex to the
bladder and lower lumbar area.

congestion, allowing normal circulation to flow through the cells as Nature intended. You can have the same results by following the directions carefully.

Case History of Bladder Trouble Healed

A woman had a weakness in her bladder and it was always giving her trouble. Sometimes it would become so bad that she would have to take to her bed. She took various medicines for the trouble which helped for a while, but it would persist in coming back after a few weeks, each time getting worse.

She decided to try reflex massage and called me to see if I would give her a course of treatments. She was not expecting it to help her, I knew by her voice on the phone, but she was coming to me as a last try for relief. This was nothing new to me as most people only try reflexology after everything else fails.

She kept her appointment and when I started to give her the treatment I found that the reflex to the pituitary was so tender that I could hardly touch her big toe. I had to hold it in the palm of my hand for a few minutes before I could even massage it. I had a hard time talking her into letting me continue with the treatment when she found out it was going to hurt.

If you find that some of the reflexes are so tender that you cannot touch them even with a "feather touch," then try holding the palm of your hand over the area for a few minutes and some of the soreness will abate enough so that you can massage it lightly at first.

I massaged the big toe lightly, then I moved on down to the thyroid reflex under the bone of the big toe. This also was very tender, and so were the adrenal reflexes in the center of her feet. In fact, all of the endocrine glands were terribly congested according to the messages the reflexes sent out. No wonder her bladder was always infected. It was a wonder she didn't have many more symptoms than that to warn her of her body being so out of harmony. She admitted that she had felt very badly for quite some time but had laid the blame on the bladder trouble. Thus the bladder is all that she had ever doctored for, when her trouble was much deeper than chronic bladder infection. It was not possible for the bladder to heal until she got to the cause of the trouble.

As I went over each reflex on her feet and explained to her what it went to and how it stimulated that certain gland with new circulation bringing it back to life, she became very interested and could even feel little shock vibrations in some of the places in her body as I massaged the reflexes to them. I didn't massage any one place on her feet more than a few seconds except the area of the bladder, as she was too full of congestion in all of the glands to take a chance of loosening too much poison into her system at once. I massaged the bladder reflex on each foot a few minutes until some of the tenderness was worked out.

She was so amazed at the improvement she felt upon getting out of the chair, that she couldn't believe it was true.

It took about five treatments in all and she never had another occurrence of bladder infection. She regained her old pep and vigor and looked and felt ten years younger within a month after starting the reflexology treatments.

CHAPTER 19

Reflexes to Sex Glands and Organs

The reflexes of the gonads or sex glands in both male and female are very important. The testes of men and the ovaries of women are associated almost exclusively with their reproductive functions. While reproduction is unquestionably the most important function of the gonads, the hormones which they produce have far-reaching effects on the body generally, and even upon mental activity.

Certain distinct cells of the ovaries and testes devote themselves to the production of steroid hormones, while others evolve into spermatozoa and ova. Both functions are closely related to and controlled by the pituitary gland.

Study Chart 3 on endocrine glands in the beginning of the book and you will see the position of the sex organs, and also the position of the reflexes to the glands. Nature has seen fit to move the reflexes to these most important glands up above the soles of the feet; maybe to protect them from overstimulation as people walked in their bare feet, as they were intended to do in the beginning of time. (See Fig. 18.)

In this area lie the reflexes to the ovaries, uterus, and fallopian tubes in the female and the testicles, penis, and prostate glands in the male.

By massaging on up the cord above the heel, a part of the sciatic nerve reflex area, the colon and rectum are also stimulated. This is understandable, since all these organs are close together in the body.

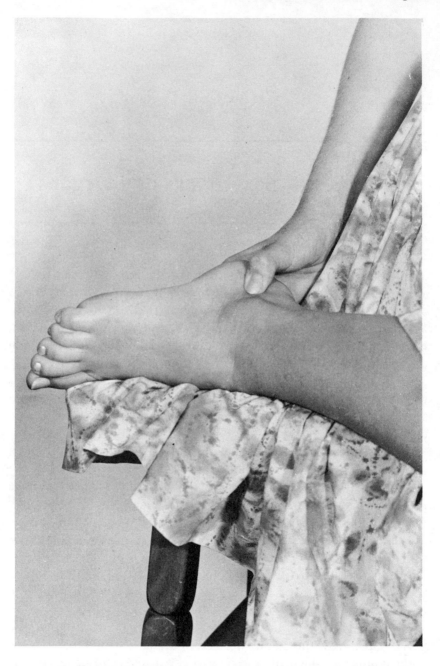

**Fig. 18. Position for massaging the reflexes to the
ovaries and testes.**

Special Techniques

On the outside of each foot, just under the ankle bone, is the reflex to the ovaries and fallopian tubes in the female and the testicles in the male. Use right foot for right side, left foot for left side.

Now by looking at Charts 3 and 4 we see that the female uterus and the male prostate and penis reflexes are found under the ankle on the inside of the foot. There will probably be some extremely tender spots in several places of this area, on both male and female, since this will cover the reflexes to all of the organs, glands, muscles, and veins in the lower section of the body that are centrally located. This is good, because when there is inflammation in any part of this area, you feel like you are one big ache, from the navel down to the lowest region. No matter what is congested, a surge of stimulation can be started by massaging the reflexes that are tender, thus equalizing the circulation and restoring health.

Look at Fig. 18 for massaging the reflexes to the ovaries and testes. Notice how the foot is pulled back and the thumb is pressed just below the ankle and above the heel bone. Or you may use the position of lifting the leg up on your lap as we have been doing, if it is more comfortable for you.

In this position, you will use the fingers to reach under the ankle to massage. Use a very gentle, rolling motion and massage this whole area under the ankle, concentrating on extremely tender spots.

This will be quite tender to most women as it involves the reflexes to the female glands, the endocrine glands (see Chart 3). I have brought relief to many pregnant women with reflexology for many different complaints, and vague aches and pains. I work on all of the reflexes, but very lightly and only one or two seconds on the area under the ankles on the inside and the outside of the feet.

Reflexes on Both Feet

Always massage reflexes on both feet — you have glands on both sides of the body; be sure and give both of them equal stimulation or you could cause poison to go from a congested ovary to a healthy one.

Massage only a few seconds the first few times that you take these treatments.

This simple reflex therapy can bring women blessed relief from many disorders which may have been troubling them for years in an amazingly short time, if the reflexes are massaged as directed here. Men also will find relief from what is, in many cases, unsuspected congestion of the gonads (sex glands).

Be persistent and faithful in massaging these reflexes, and you will enjoy the results of Nature's wonderful healing forces being summoned to deal with an unhealthy situation.

Sex Organ Reflex Techniques

Take the foot up into position for massaging. See Fig. 19, "Reflexes to the uterus, penis, and prostate." Notice how the thumb of the right hand presses between the ankle and the heel on the inside of the left foot.

Now, press firmly with a rolling motion of the thumb, moving back and forth, being sure to cover the entire area under the ankle. Give special attention to the very tender places, keeping in mind that some of these reflexes are tiny, pinpoint spots and the area must be covered thoroughly.

For some, it may be easier to use the right hand to massage the left foot, and others to use the right hand to massage the right foot. Do whichever is easier for you. And remember *do not overmassage* the first few times; just a few seconds on each reflex, and Nature will do her part in her good time.

One needs to know that these sex glands and organs are not only for the purpose of reproduction of new life, but they have a much more important role in the body, that of regeneration of the whole body of which they are a part.

Sex Gland Functions

The genital gland has a dual function. Testicles, for instance, secrete spermatozoa, the motile generative element of the semen, externally. But they also secrete internally substances such as hormones which affect not only the sexual characteristics, but the

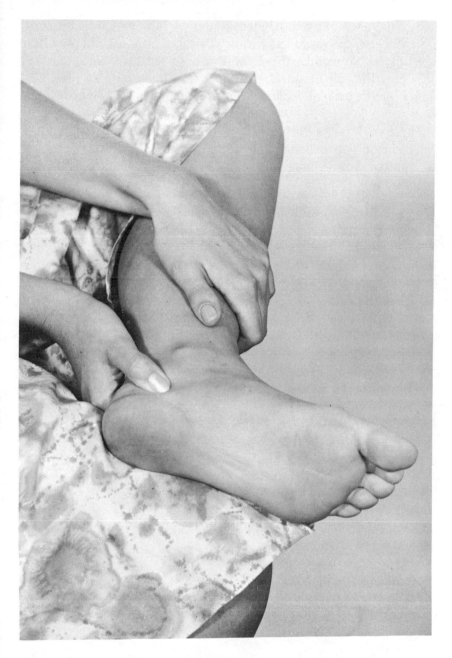

Fig. 19. Position for massaging the reflexes to the
uterus, penis, and prostate gland.

body as a whole, as well as mental and personality characteristics.

No organ can keep its vitality without stimulation by these substances. No wonder these glands are so sensitive, since they not only play the role of starting life in a new body (a baby), but also they keep the cells of our own organs young, healthy, vigorous, and vital.

These organs play a big part in the rejuvenation of our bodies. Never neglect to massage the reflexes to these glands and organs, no matter how young or old you are. Stagnation is *death;* circulation is *LIFE!*

CHAPTER 20

Reflexes to Prostate Gland

The prostate gland is the largest accessory male sex structure, encircling the neck of the urethra (outlet tube for urine) as it emerges from the bladder. The prostate is a broad, fore-shortened, heart-shaped organ, composed of mucus-secreting glands.

Functions of the Prostate Gland

The prostate lies immediately in front of the rectum, so the reflexes will be the same for the prostate as for the rectum. The prostate neutralizes the acid suspension of sperm, increasing the likelihood of fertilization for reproduction purposes. It is not absolutely essential that the prostate be intact, and because it does not secrete hormones, it is relatively dispensable.

Secretions of the prostate collect in several ducts which emerge into the urethra through a common hillock. Secretion is continuous, with periodic excretion into the urine. You can see what happens if circulation to this gland is slowed down and congestion results. The flow of secretion from the ducts into the urine will be slowed down, and in time the ducts would become swollen and inflamed from congestion.

An enlargement of the prostate will result in a great deal of difficulty in voiding the urine, causing the patient to urinate often, suffer considerable pain, and experience other bodily complaints.

Benefits of Prostate Reflex Conditioning

The prostate is another gland that can cause so much suffering in men, in some cases for years; yet it is so simple and easy to bring it back to health by massaging the prostate reflexes. I brought complete relief to every case I have ever treated, and in many cases only two or three treatments were needed to start the normal circulation back into the inflamed and enlarged glands.

Special Prostate Reflex Technique

Let us get into position to massage the reflexes to the prostate, which will be in the same location on both feet. We will use the illustration for massaging the reflex to the prostate (Fig. 19 , page 111). The thumb is pressing on the prostate reflex; notice how the thumb of the hand presses between the ankle and the heel on the inside of the foot . You may use the knuckle of the forefinger, the Reflex Hand Massager, or a like device to press in and rotate gently with a rolling massage. If you have the right leg in position, you will use the left hand for massaging this reflex. Be sure you massage both feet.

Prostate Trouble Gives No Advance Publicity

Many times prostate trouble starts in young men and slowly advances without their ever being conscious of its increasing danger, until the gland becomes congested enough to cause them discomfort and pain.

I have discovered many congested prostate glands in men that came to me for other complaints. The congestion was not to the extent that it had caused any adverse symptoms as yet so the patients were not aware that it was there. This is so true of many diseases; they creep up on us slowly and secretly until they are well established, and then they strike us suddenly. This is the wonderful magic of reflexology: it not only helps Nature maintain a free-flowing circulation so that she can renew sick and worn-out cells, but it helps her send a surge of stimulating, life-giving circulation throughout every cell in the body so that congestion will not have a chance to build up for a sneak attack in the future.

Cases of Prostate Healing

One elderly man, Mr. B., came to me as a last hope for relief of prostate troubles. He hadn't had a good night's sleep in three months because of having to get up so often to urinate, and from the discomfort of the enlarged gland. He was extremely nervous, as this complaint does affect the nervous system.

I was surprised to find a man of his age in such fine health, as the only tender place on his feet was the one leading to the prostate. When I remarked about this, he said that otherwise he did enjoy perfect health. The prostate reflexes were extremely tender, and I had to use very little pressure at first. After massaging only a few moments he remarked that he felt quite relaxed and that the pressure seemed much less. When Mr. B. returned for his second treatment two days later, he was very happy to tell me that he had slept like a baby all night through, didn't have to get up during the night anymore, and felt much better. I noted when I massaged the reflexes for the second time that most of the tenderness was gone. He went back home the next day, and his daughter says he is still doing fine.

His perfect health condition, other than the congested prostate, probably was a factor in his quick recovery. But after reading this, you men need not suffer needlessly from a faulty prostate gland, ever. You know how to handle the situation now.

How a Stubborn Case of "Prostate" Was Healed

When Mr. F. called my office for an appointment he said he thought his problem was "prostate trouble." I assured him that we had gotten almost unbelievable results on this condition with reflexology.

When Mr. F. was seated in the chair, and I had his feet in my hands, I started with the big toe, looking for a tender spot in the center which would tell me what condition the pituitary gland was in before I tried any other reflexes. I found a tremendous response to massage in the center of the big toe, as I had expected if the prostate was not functioning properly. Next, I moved on down the foot, pressing and searching for other "messages" that the reflexes could give me pertaining to his condition.

As I massaged, Mr. F. told me of the symptoms of distress. He was subject to spells of illness if he overworked, or if he ate certain foods such as asparagus, of which he was so fond that he had a large garden full of it. The whole lower region of the abdomen would become sore and "tight" as if everything from his waist down were inflamed. He would become quite ill and have to remain in bed for several days at a time with hardly any food. Doctors had suggested that it might be prostate gland trouble. They had given him treatment for it which had not helped, and as he grew older, each episode seemed more severe.

As I started to massage under the ankle bone, I found that the reflexes to the testes were much more tender than the ones to the prostate. When I told him so, he said that when he was quite young, he had been injured by a fall with a horse and that the doctors had to remove one of the testes, but he had never had any trouble from the other one so far as he could tell.

I found the reflexes to both of the testes so tender that I could barely touch them. The reflex on the left foot was worse than the one on the right; and since the right testis had been removed, the tender reflex to it was an indication of scar tissue. You will find this true in any case of an operation or injury. The reflexes will always tell you if there is an obstruction or constriction, and even though scar tissue is necessary to mend an operation site, injury, or serious infection, it can develop into a health problem. Sometimes it is necessary to remove it by surgery.

The claim that massaging these reflexes can dissolve irritating scar tissue may sound like a pretty bold statement, but if doctors were correct in their diagnoses in some of the cases I have worked on, there is ample evidence to show that reflex massage does alleviate the distress.

In the case of Mr. F., the reflex to the testis on the left foot was much more tender than the one on the right, which indicated that the root of his problem probably was in the left testis. I did not find any of the other reflexes in either foot nearly as tender at those under the ankles on the outside of the feet. If his real trouble had been from the prostate, then the reflexes on the inner side of the feet would have given the pain signal when pressed and massaged.

I concentrated mainly on the reflex to the pituitary in the big toe; also the pineal which has its reflex in the big toe, a little to the side of the location of the pituitary; then to the adrenal reflexes located in the center of the foot just over the kidney area.

Now, take warning here again — note that I was careful not to massage these reflexes for over five seconds on each foot for the first few treatments, because they cannot be massaged without also massaging the kidney reflexes. For this reason, a few seconds is all that you must use on this area until most of the tenderness is worked out. This should only take three or four reflex applications.

Mr. F. said he felt so much relief and so relaxed after the first treatment that he wanted to come back in two days. He came faithfully for two weeks, even though nearly all of his adverse and painful symptoms had vanished after the third treatment.

CHAPTER 21

Reflex Relief for Hemorrhoids

Hemorrhoids are nothing more than congested veins (known as piles). These are actually varicose veins in the rectum. They can become so large as to protrude, causing inconvenience, much suffering, and in many cases excessive bleeding.

They are one of the most painful diseases and usually are suffered in silence by those who have them; yet with reflex massage they are one of the quickest to respond to treatment, at least where pain is concerned. This chapter on hemorrhoids is written for those who have been suffering from them for many years in silent pain.

Reflex Techniques

Here we will learn how to use the reflexology method to bring you prompt relief. Lift your leg up into position for massage; see Fig. 20 for massaging the reflexes for hemorrhoids. It doesn't make any difference which foot you use first, as both of them will have to be massaged. You may find one more tender than the other when you get started, and, of course, it will be massaged the most. Notice also on Chart 4, the cord up the back of the leg and the outer edge of the heel where you find the hemorrhoid reflexes.

If you are using the Rollo Massager here, it will work very nicely on the cord on the back of the leg, but you will probably have to find the tender reflex on the edge of the heel with the thumb or fingers in a press and feel method. If you have the right foot in

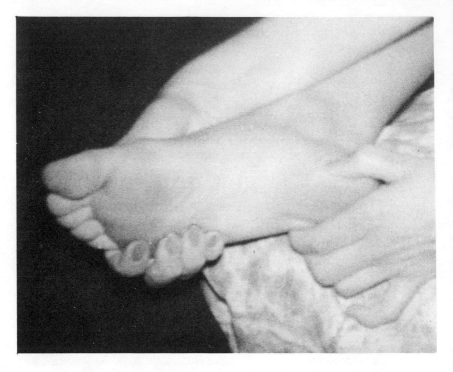

Fig. 20. Position for massaging the reflexes for he-morrhoids.

position, then use the left hand for massaging as shown in Fig. 20. In this massage you will use a different motion; instead of rolling with the thumb it is better to press on the bony edge of the heel and press downward toward the heel pad with a firm pulling down motion. Go all the way around the heel, using the thumb on one side and the forefinger on the other side, whichever is the most convenient for you to work with the most pressure.

The tender reflex may only cover the area of a small bean, but you will know it when you press it. That will probably be the reflex to the congested vein in the rectum which is causing all the trouble. Sometimes there is just one spot and then there may be several. You will soon learn where these are and be able to find them immediately when pain strikes. If you have trouble finding the spot, keep pressing and moving the fingers back and forth, and press in deeper until you do find it. It is there!

Massaging the Cord

Then let us massage the cord on the back of the leg, starting just above the heel as shown on Chart 4. The best way to massage this reflex is to put the thumb on one side of the cord and the fingers on the other side and massage it up and down from the heel to where it disappears into the calf of the leg. This area can sometimes be unbearably tender and you will have to start with a "feather touch," increasing the pressure as the tenderness diminishes. Remember, this area contains the reflexes to all of the lower region of the body, such as the prostate and gonad glands. It also stimulates the lower lumbar region.

Bend the foot as far back as possible, stretching the cord and massaging it in this position a few moments; then stretch the foot out as far as possible and again massage the cord. We want this cord to become limber and relaxed, which may take some time to accomplish. The tenderness may be very severe and you will think you can't stand the pain, but the result will be worth the "torture," as some call it. Remember, as the tenderness gradually works out, the condition will improve. The more the pain, the more the inflammation in that area.

Another condition which can cause untold agony is a prolapsed rectum, and as a person gets older, this will probably become worse, protruding more and more. It is very often badly swollen and very much inflamed. The benefits and results are almost unbelievable for this serious form of trouble when reflex massage is used. You will use the same method which you used for the hemorrhoid and rectum disorders. Don't let the simplicity of reflex massage rob it of its importance in healing.

CHAPTER 22

Reflex to the Sciatic Nerve

The great sciatic nerve is the largest nerve cord in the body, measuring three-quarters of an inch in breadth. It passes out of the pelvis and descends along the back part of the thigh to about its lower third where it divides into two large branches. It supplies nearly the whole of the integument of the leg, the muscles of the back of the thigh, and those of the leg and foot.

When there is inflammation of the sciatic nerve, one is in for much pain. Many people suffer for years without getting any relief. I believe that I have treated more cases of leg aches than any other malady, and most of them were caused by inflammation of the sciatic nerve.

There can be several reasons for this nerve causing such intense pain; an injury to some other part of the body, an enlarged prostate gland, constipation, and many times a misplacement in the lower spine, will result in the torture of sciatica.

You can readily see the agony that one goes through when inflammation has slowed down the circulation of this large nerve that affects almost the whole lower part of the body. Yet it is so amazingly simple to banish all inflammation from this great nerve in an unbelievably short time by massaging the reflexes to it.

Reflex Techniques

Let us lift the leg into position. If you have aches and pains in one leg, let us start on it. Lift it up into the position for massaging.

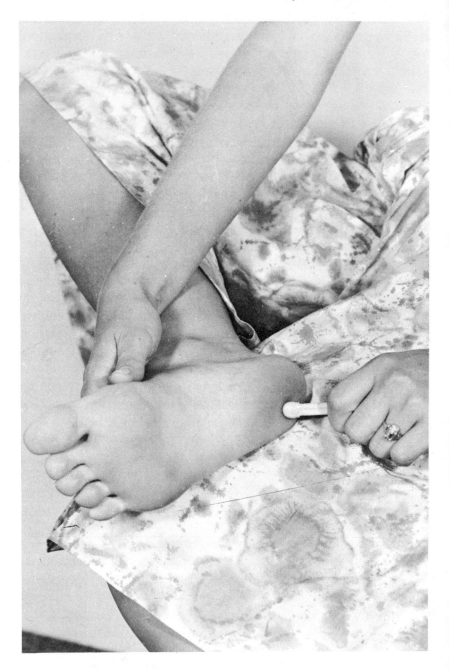

Fig. 21. Position for massaging the reflex to the sciatic nerve, using the hand Reflex Massager.

(See illustration for massaging sciatic reflexes, Fig. 21, and notice that the hand Reflex Massager is being used here.)

It is doubtful that you can reach this particular reflex with the thumb or knuckle unless it is extremely tender; then it would be difficult to massage with enough pressure to pulverize the crystals causing the congestion. Because the reflex is usually quite deep, take the massager or other device in your hand and press it into the bottom of the heel, as in the picture. The reflex will be found almost, but not quite, in the center of the heel pad, a little back from the center and toward the outside of the foot (notice position in illustration). The way to find the exact spot is to use the press and feel method. If you are pressing hard enough, you will know when you find the reflex button because of intense pain.

The treatment is better if it can be done with no covering on the legs, especially silk or rayon. Always massage the reflexes on both feet, and both legs.

Sciatic Nerve Pointers

Now, having found the spot, massage it with a deep, rolling motion. At first it may be so tender that it brings tears to your eyes. Relax the pressure a little as the pain subsides. In many cases the massaging of the reflex to the end of this great nerve has brought complete relief from leg aches in one treatment. Yours may take several treatments — it also could be healed with one treatment. If it works for others it will work for you, if you follow the directions and use them faithfully for one treatment or six, until the torture of persistent leg aches stop. They will if the pains are caused by a congested sciatic nerve. Massage only a few moments at first.

We have just massaged the ending of the sciatic nerve. Now let us move on up to the inner side of the ankle bone where the nerve lies nearest the surface. With the thumb, press above and back of the ankle. You will probably experience intense pain in this area but not from the sciatic nerve alone. As you can see from Chart 4, this covers reflexes to most of the lower extremities of the body. When you are massaging this area, you are sending the healing forces of Nature to all inflamed and congested parts in the lower lumbar region. Massage this area with a pressing, rolling motion.

Working Up to the Knee Area

Keeping the same position, in back of the ankle, you will massage on up the inside of the leg, working up the bone until you come to the knee. You will come across several places that are more tender than others; massage these a few seconds, then continue on to the next tender spot. These are like signal buttons buried under the skin. Touch one and it flashes a pain signal telling that there is trouble in the circulation line — so work it out. The Rollo Reflex Massager may be used for easier massaging of this area. Massage slowly and gently all the way to the knee. The number of sore spots will come as a surprise, especially around the knee area. Always the massage should be gentle, but with the massager or fingers pressing in as deeply as the tenderness will permit.

When you have found and massaged the tender spots of the knee, with the thumb of the same hand as the leg you are massaging, move just above the knee and continue the press and roll, massaging on up the inside of the leg (thigh) until you can feel the tenderness subside, almost to the groin.

Next do the same progressive massage up the outside of the leg, starting at the back of the ankle bone, ending at the knee. This stimulates circulation in the legs, banishes congestion, and brings blessed relief from many leg troubles.

An Additional Reflex from the Back

We will go on to massage one more reflex to the sciatic nerve. Reach around to the back a little below the waistline, put your fingers on your spine, about 1 or 2 inches up from your tailbone or end of the spine. Now move the fingers toward the front of the body about the width of the hand where you can feel the movement of the joint of the upper leg. Press in and around this joint with thumb or finger until a severe pain is felt, or at least a sore spot. There again the method must be press and feel for the signal button. When it is located, wonders can be accomplished for healing the sciatic nerve by the simple process of pressing on it with the finger, not hard, but holding it as long as the pressure is endurable — like holding in the button on a doorbell.

If you have gotten the correct position, the sensation will be like that caused by a hot poker being thrust in there.

Reflex Area Back of Ankle

Next massage the whole area along the cord in back of the ankle.

Follow that with a massage of the entire area above the heel and along the cord at the back of the leg on both sides, as you would for prostate, hemorrhoids, and the lower lumbar region.

A Case of Sciatic Healing

Mr. M, a college professor and Naval Reserve Officer, came to me with a terrible pain in his heel. He had run the gauntlet of Navy hospitals and private doctors where the only thing they did for him, he said, was to give him deadening shots in the heel which would last at the most three hours — and the condition was becoming worse. He came to me without any faith, but at the insistence of his wife and neighbors. When I told him I thought I knew what was the matter with him, he seemed quite surprised.

When I pressed into the sciatic nerve reflex in the bottom of his heel, he nearly jumped out of the chair with pain. "That is it!" he said. He was amazed at the almost instant relief, and after only one more treatment never had a recurrence of sciatic trouble. If you don't get such gratifying results in three days, remember persistent effort and a little patience will accomplish the desired results.

CHAPTER 23

Reflex to Condition the Lymph Glands

Throughout the body there is an extensive network which carries lymph. The lymph vessels collect fluids which have seeped through the blood vessels' walls, and return them to the bloodstream via two main lymphatic ducts, emptying into two subclavian veins near the heart. The lymph nodes (glands) — enlarged tissue masses in the lymph vessels — are filtering devices for removing dead cells and other foreign matter.

What Lymph Glands Do

The lymph nodes near the lungs are black, because the lymph from the lungs carry out the dust we breathe. When a finger is infected, the many lymph nodes in the armpit may become swollen and tender as the lymph drains bacteria into this spot. If there is infection on the foot, there may be a swelling of the lymph nodes in the groin of the leg. Lymph nodes are protective in many ways. They destroy infection. At frequent intervals the lymph channels enter and emerge from these lymph nodes or glands.

Nature placed a lot of these little seedlike nodes in the neck to safeguard against infection from the tonsils, teeth, etc.

It is estimated that the body has some 600 to 700 of these tiny nodes. Their importance is realized at once, and also the need to give them proper stimulation.

Let us now look at Fig. 22 for the position to massage the

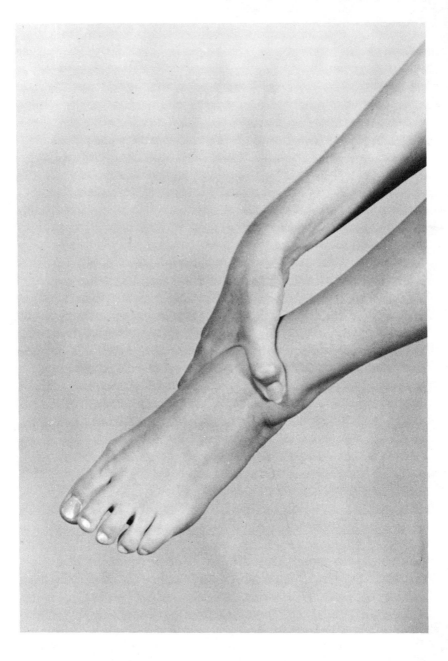

Fig. 22. Position for massaging the reflexes to the lymph glands.

reflexes to these many lymph glands.

Notice how the thumb is curled over the top of the foot just above the ankle. This pretty well covers the location of the lymph reflexes on the feet. The whole area on top of the foot is to be massaged, from outside ankle bone to inside ankle bone, holding the fingers just above the ankle bones. There are several positions that may be used to massage these reflexes to the lymph glands; use the one that is easiest and most natural for you.

In Fig. 22 we see the thumb being used, curling across the whole area on top of the foot. You will use the whole thumb instead of just the end of it in this particular massage, since we are not trying to massage a single reflex but many of them. Roll the whole thumb over the area in a circular motion, pressing in as you progress.

You may find the simplest way to massage these lymph reflexes is to put the left leg up into position on the lap and grasp the inside of the top of the left foot, above the ankle bones, with the left hand thumb to the inside of the foot. Now, with the first finger curling over the top of the foot, massage the whole area at once with the whole finger pressing and rolling as you progress back and forth between and just above the ankle bones, wherever you find it is tender. You have many glands to cover here in this small area, Remember, if it hurts, massage it. You will find the fingers fit very naturally over the curve of the foot and the massaging is easy to do. Do the right foot the same way, being sure to massage the reflexes on both feet always.

CHAPTER 24

How to Condition Reflexes for General Rejuvenation

How old is old? Most people think that their normal life span is "three score years and ten" and if they live beyond the age of 70, they are living on borrowed time.

Would you like to be young again? No, not really! You would not like to part with the knowledge you have gained through the long years of trial and error. But you would like to walk expectantly into the future, to enjoy new experiences, with a revitalized body, wouldn't you? We all would! People say, "If I could just be young again, and know what I know now."

We can do nothing about our chronological age; but we do not have to feel old — or be old — at the age of 70 or beyond.

According to Dr. Andrew von Salza, a specialist in rejuvenation, "To rejuvenate the body while the mind is saturated with thoughts of senility would not be effective." On the other hand, to expect a healthy mind to produce a healthy body without providing necessary elements conducive to youth would likewise be a fallacy.

Dr. von Salza recommends thinking young to those who feel like senile derelicts. Each person should start a program to prevent senility as a personal task, since at the present time no one is immune to becoming a senile derelict — if he lives long enough.

Dr. von Salza goes on to say quite frequently one becomes a senile derelict overnight — even though senility is not prepared overnight.

"It is prepared," he says, "through years of neglect of the body." Your body is just as strong as its weakest part. What are your weak points? Tiring easily, slips of memory, wrinkles, difficulty getting up from a chair?

Start to rejuvenate yourself before even such signs develop, because when they do develop, your body is sounding an alarm.

Listen for these signals better than you listen to noises in your car. You can buy a new car, but not a new body.

Since time immemorial people have been looking for means of rejuvenation outside of themselves, the search for the "Fountain of Youth," rejuvenation through witchcraft, etc. The only place where there are such possibilities is within yourself.

Drs. Steinach and Voronoff sought possibilities of bodily rejuvenation by means of rejuvenating the genital glands.

Through various therapies it is possible to revive glandular vitality in such a measure that the body will be put on the path to reactivate its natural process of rejuvenation — adequate regeneration and growth of cells. Through various therapies the body can be provided with the necessary materials and the will to rebuild itself, mainly in the genital glands.

Ann Walsh writes of her experience in taking estrogen replacement therapy. She says, "What happened after I had been taking my pills for a while was like waking from a bad dream. I felt like a woman again, a well woman, a much younger woman." Estrogen is a hormone replacement.

According to Doctor Davis, when a woman's ovaries no longer supply her with estrogen (the hormone supplied by the ovaries), at menopause she begins to age. She has back and joint pains, loss of height, high blood pressure, drying and shrinking of the vaginal lining, loss of skin tone and body firmness, and osteoporosis (fragility and porousness of the bones) — a disorder of the skeleton that results in fractures of the hip, shoulder, wrist, and spine. Osteoporosis occurs in about 25 per cent of women within five to ten years following "change of life." Estrogen replacement retards osteoporosis by reversing the process of calcium wastage from the bones.

Male and Female Hormones

A man does not develop osteoporosis until he becomes senile, because he is getting androgens (male hormones) from his testes as long as he lives. There are two factors in maintaining the bony skeleton. One of them is estrogens in women and androgens in men. The other factor is activity. This is extremely important, according to Dr. Davis.

Hot flashes play an important part of the post-menopause in women. They age more rapidly; insomnia and nervousness are frequent complaints. Liver metabolism, bone development, skin tissue changes, and particularly heart and blood vessel diseases are laid to the lack of estrogen hormones.

What are those mysterious substances which are the active principles of regeneration?

Science has discovered various therapies to revive glandular vitality so as to reactivate their natural processes of rejuvenation. There is the ovary-produced hormone, estrogen, artificially produced and given to women with wonderfully blessed results; also there is the rejuvenation through live cell therapy, perfected by Dr. von Salza.

How to make Reflexology Your Rejuvenator

Now we come to reflexology, the scientific massage of the reflexes to stimulate normal circulation by relieving congestion in the various nerve endings in the hands and the feet.

I could tell you of so many cases, but I will tell you of the one concerning post-menopause, since this is the main factor of aging in women.

A Case of "Hot Flashes" Healed

Mrs. M. called me and asked what I could do for hot flashes. She was having them so bad that she had to go to bed at times. The shots the doctors gave her only lasted a few hours and sometimes did not even bring relief. She was desperate as she had to work to support her family.

Since reflex massage stimulates the circulation of every gland in the body, I told her to come and see what results we would get. Mrs. M. felt better in the first few minutes of massaging the reflexes. When she came for her second treatment in two days she was elated. She had gone home and slept like a baby the whole night; she had been free of hot flashes for two days and was just beginning to feel light ones starting again. She felt a new surge of energy, a spiritual uplift, a new zest for life. She did not need very many treatments, and as long as I knew her the symptoms never returned. This is worth careful consideration.

How the Reflexes Worked to Rejuvenate

By massaging the reflex to the ovaries, I stimulated a normal production of the hormone, estrogen. By massaging the reflex to the pituitary gland and relieving congestion, those hormones were put back into circulation. Her natural body rebuilding process had started to slow down. With reflexology I put the process in reverse by stimulating the endocrine glands so that they were able to produce and pour into the cellulary system certain substances which regulate the metabolic processes, growth, and morphology of cells. This we must have to keep young.

So long as the rebuilding of cells is adequate, the organism is young. As soon as this rebuilding process starts to slow down, the organism is getting old — and so are you!

A Case of Senility Helped

I also rejuvenated my ailing, senile, 85-year-old mother, treating her myself after taking her out of the hospital. She became a pleasant, happy companion for many years.

Let us learn to give the stimulating massage that will bring relaxation to the entire body. (See Fig. 23 for relieving body tension.)

To do this, take the foot up on the lap as shown in the picture. Take the end of the foot in the opposite hand and with a rolling motion, twist the whole foot. Roll the foot in as large a circle as you can. Don't force it; just roll it gently around and around, twisting as you roll (note Fig. 23). This will relax the tenseness of the whole body, as if someone were giving you a body massage. If the foot seems stiff and tense, then your body is in a like condition. After you have limbered the foot up a bit, reverse the rolling procedure and roll it in the opposite direction; then change feet,

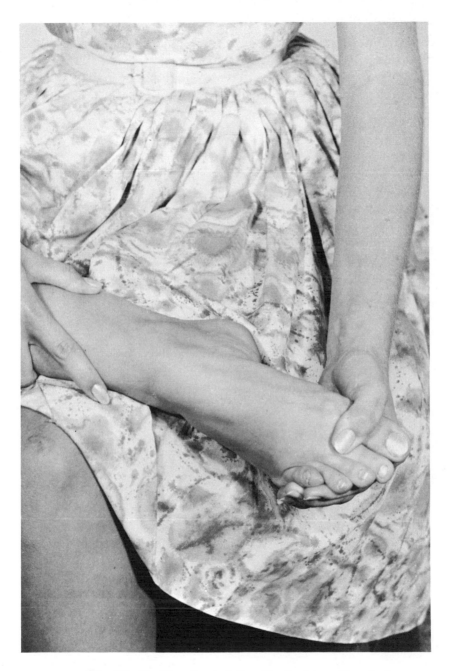

Fig. 23. Position for twisting the foot to relieve body tension.

using the same procedure. I find it is good to start out with a few seconds of this relaxing massage at the beginning of the treatments, and then use it again at the end of massaging.

I have proved this scientific method of healing beyond a doubt in my experience. Try it on yourself and *feel* the beneficial results.

CHAPTER 25

How Reflexology Helps Health of All Glands

Every cell in the human body is capable of being energized by the substances emitted from the endocrine glands, the seven centers of vital force which act as electrical battery storages for the purpose of constantly recreating life.

Therefore, a major requisite for a perfect body is to have the cellular tissue mineralized, vitaminized, and hence ionized to receive these emanations. Minerals and vitamins must be absorbed into the bloodstream, the vitamins bringing the otherwise dead minerals to life.

The Glands as Watchdogs of the Body

The glands have been aptly termed the watchdogs of the body. They trap the necessary nutriments, and, in conjunction with their internal secretions, form them into powerful crystallizations, much as the essences of flowers are mixed with the internal secretions of the bees to be converted into honey.

These crystallizations have been given the name of hormones. These influence all the activities of life. An example would be a deficiency of the thyroid secretion, which would prevent the natural growth of the body and interfere with the rhythmical functioning of the heart.

A deficiency of the sex hormone would cause sterility and other sex maladjustments, and since there is a close affinity between the complete circle of glands, it is liable to affect the whole behavior of the person thus afflicted.

It has been claimed that the hormones send out particles of material substances into the bloodstream. Others maintain that this is not so, declaring the hormones send out radio-electric emanations which have been generated in the glandular pow-erhouses. The radiant waves travel along the cerebro-nervous system, which, when it is tuned to a high state of efficiency, broadcasts waves of energy to the remotest cell in the body. When the waves are not powerful enough, millions of cells are left dormant or stagnant. This is the start of disease, for when too many cells die, the body is reduced to a state of autointoxication.

What Tiredness Indicates

Actually, a feeling of tiredness is an announcement that the generators of the electric charges are not functioning at the optimum of their efficiency. Further investigation will reveal that there is either a mineral or a vitamin deficiency in the bloodstream.

It has already been established what can be done by touching off the spark by reflex massage of the feet.

The Seven Endocrine Gland Watchdogs

Let us look, then at these seven watchdogs, the endocrine glands. These are often identified as the ductless glands because they have no ducts and secrete their hormones directly into the bloodstream. Thus there is what is called the endocrine system which is comprised of the pituitary and pineal glands, situated in the cavity of the skull; the thyroid and parathyroids near the larynx at the base of the neck; the thymus which lies in the chest above the heart; the pair of adrenals placed atop the kidneys like two little hoods; and the gonads, the sex glands.

These so-called ductless glands cooperate in determining the forms of our bodies and the workings of our minds. They are all closely interrelated and supplement and depend on each other.

Every individual owes his development and well-being to the normal functions of these glands. The minute secretions called hormones sent into the bloodstream by these glands are responsible for the difference between a genius and an imbecile, between a dwarf and a giant, a person who is happy and one who is cheerless.

The potency of the endocrine glands is beyond comprehension. They control our activity, energy, stabilization, radiance, mobility, and organization of life processes.

They are also the main glands that the reflexes will stimulate to a normal functioning, and that herbs nourish with their wealth of vitamins and minerals.

It is very likely that much of the synthetic medicines put into the blood are responsible for the malfunctioning of one or the other of these glands, and they do have to work in perfect harmony with each other or all sorts of ailments occur in the body.

The Rewards of Harmonizing Your Gland Activities

Learning to so live that the endocrine glands harmonize will, in turn, enable you to live with a sound body and vibrant health. You will find your illnesses inclined to vanish. The secret is to stimulate each of them in every natural way available.

Pituitary Gland

The diagram of the endocrine glands (Chart 3) in this book shows that most important pituitary gland located at the base of the brain just at the midpoint of the head, as though carefully hidden in the safest and most inaccessible place — and well it should be, as it is vastly needed. Although it is only about 1/40th of an ounce, it has the biggest job to do, that of keeping the other glands in harmony with each other. Its task could be compared to that of first violin, on which a great orchestra depends!

The pituitary gland controls the inner mobility and agility of the system, promoting the proper growth of the body, glands, and organs, including sexual development. It maintains the efficiency of the various structures and prevents the excessive accumulation of fat. A relaxed, harmonious, and happy person, without complexes and frustrations, is sure to possess a normal, healthy, and active pituitary gland.

And remember the reflexes for the pituitary are located in the center of each big toe.

Pineal Gland

It will be noted that the pineal gland lies quite close to the pituitary with the same treatments generally used for it; reflexes being a little to the side of the center of the big toe.

It has been established that a pathological condition of this gland strongly influences the sex glands, causing premature development of the entire system.

It acts with the body as a sort of organizer, or harmonizer, controlling the development of the glands and keeping them in proper range. The pineal gland's normal activity keeps the functions of the endocrine system harmonious and effective.

This gland is even smaller than the pituitary, but is quite important to one's well-being!

It is known that the pituitary gland secretes hormones into the bloodstream. The pituitary actually is divided into two parts, or it might be said, two separate glands, the rear section called the posterior lobe and the forward portion the anterior lobe. Both lobes produce polypeptide hormones. The anterior lobe produces six hormones that have been definitely isolated as pure, or nearly pure, substances. The existence of several other hormones is suspected.

Of the six hormones, one has been found to have the function of stimulating the thyroid gland. Removal of the pituitary gland in experimental animals caused atrophy of the thyroid gland and many other unpleasant effects. Thus, it can be seen how important it is to keep these glands stimulated with reflexology and in perfect working order.

Since these first two endocrine glands have such an influence on the thyroid, let's see what importance it has on body and mind.

Thyroid Gland

The thyroid is a soft mass of yellowish-red, glandular tissue about 2 inches high and slightly more than 2 inches wide, weighing an ounce or less. It exists in two lobes, one on either side of the windpipe with a narrow, connecting band running in front of the windpipe just at the bottom of what is commonly known as the Adam's apple. See Chart 3.

Thyroid conditions, so far, are treated with iodine. The best analyses at present show that the human thyroid at most contains 8 milligrams, (or about 1/2000th of an ounce) of iodine. The iodine concentration in the thyroid gland is more than 60,000 times as high as is the concentration anywhere else in the body.

Years ago, the fact that iodine was present in such minute quantities made it seem unimportant, because at that time, such things as essential trace elements were unknown. Now we have learned that elements form parts of hormones or enzymes, and are necessary to proper functioning of the body and even life itself, without having to be present in more than these extremely small quantities.

The richest source of iodine in natural form is from the sea. Seaweed is the best, because plant cells actively concentrate the iodine of the sea. Marine life is rich in iodine. There is a hormone produced by the thyroid gland which is called thyroglobulin which contains iodine from which small fragments of the thyroglobulin molecule are passed off into the bloodstream.

Then there is the thyroid hormone thyroxine, and tri-iodothyronine. These are made up of carbon, hydrogen, nitrogen, and oxygen.

There are many questions yet to be answered concerning the thyroid and its hormones in medical science.

Exactly what is the importance of the thyroid gland, and what is its influence on the body?

The degree of thyroid activity makes one either alert or dull, quick or slow, animated or depressed, mentally keen or apathetic. It is also responsible for the inner activity of one's system, preventing the retention of water, sluggishness of the tissues, and densification of the bones.

Proper development of and functioning of the sex organs also depend upon the healthy and normal functioning of the thyroid.

This is the gland which, having become enlarged, is called goiter. Since the knowledge of iodine's use, this trouble is seldom encountered any more.

The reflex to the thyroid is down from the big toe and under the large toe bone to the center of the foot ever so little. Massage of the entire area is important, from just under the toe down to the inner edge of the foot.

Any seeming difficulty with the thyroid is quite possibly caused by a malfunctioning of the pituitary which is affecting this gland.

Parathyroid Glands

Behind the thyroid gland lie four flattened scraps of pinkish-reddish tissue, each about one-third of an inch long. Two are on either side of the windpipe, one of each pair being near the top of the thyroid and one near the bottom. These are the parathyroid glands, shown in Chart 3.

These glands influence the stability within the body, the maintenance of its metabolic equilibrium, by controlling the distribution and activity of calcium and phosphorus in the system.

The calcium is essential to blood coagulation, and to the proper working of nerve and muscle. To do its work properly, calcium must remain within a narrow range of concentration. Should it rise too high or drop too low, the entire ion balance of the blood is upset. Neither nerves nor muscles can do their work; and the body through a failure in organization, dies. It is the proper functioning of the parathyroid gland which keeps this from happening. Poise and tranquility are the results of the normal function of these glands.

The reflexes will be the same as for the thyroid, except there appears to be a need for *deeper* massage. Press slightly harder in the area of the thyroid, massaging back behind it, careful not to bruise the tissue or capillaries.

Thymus Gland

We are born with the thymus gland lying in the upper chest in front of the lungs and above the heart, just below the thyroid gland, as shown in Chart 3. It extends upward into the neck.

In children the thymus is soft and pink, with mazy lobes. It is fairly large, weighing as much as 40 grams or 1½ ounces.

As puberty is reached, the gland diminishes in importance as well as in size.

As the age of 13 or 14 arrives, the child awakens from his dream life into reality. The thymus gland must shrink or the adjustment between man and earth would be retarded and could even cause death.

To massage the reflexes of the thymus gland, work close to those for the thyroid again, a little to the center of the foot and the area just below the thyroid reflex.

As long as the other endocrine glands are kept in harmony with each other, there is no occasion to be concerned about the thymus.

Adrenal Glands

The adrenal glands, small caps astride the kidneys, influence our entire activities, our vigor, courage, and fervor expressed in every way. They promote the inner drive to action, keenness of perception, untiring activity.

They are sometimes referred to as the fight or flight glands. Under pressure of strong emotion, the gland releases two hormones, adrenalin and noradrenalin which have an immediate and profound effect on the machinery of the body, mobilizing its resources for a state of emergency. Heartbeat is accelerated, circulation is increased, blood sugar level rises. The adrenalin hormone stimulates fear while the noradrenalin hormone tends to make one angry and ready to fight.

It is a fairly well-established fact that the timid, introverted, neurotic type of person possesses adrenal glands which are not producing a sufficient amount of noradrenalin, and too large an amount of adrenalin. It is contended that this results from insufficient support, causing degeneration of the glands coupled partly with disturbances within the blood sugar regulating mechanism.

It is now necessary to come back to the pituitary gland for help, as the adrenal and it accomplish their functions in controlling blood-sugar level in this way. When the blood-sugar level starts to dip below normal limits, the pituitary gets busy and secretes what is called ACTH into the blood. This is picked up by the adrenal and stimulates the gland into secreting cortisone and cortin into the blood. These adrenal hormones, in turn, cause the liver, as well as the body's muscles, to give up some of their stored body sugar.

Through the action of the pancreatic product, glucagon is released and changed into soluble glucose, the blood form of sugar. This process takes place until the blood's sugar is up to a normal level.

If the adrenal glands were permitted to lose their efficiency or become impaired in function, the body would be in for serious trouble, and probably the mind as well, since the brain must have a constant supply of sugar at all times or it will become critically damaged.

It must be kept in mind that the glands make this blood sugar out of the foods eaten. Commercial sugars are not referred to here, but rather, use of Nature's sugars such as are found in fruits and vegetables.

Here again, medical science has many questions still unanswered in the entire physical-chemical spectrum. But in treating any and all parts of the body with Nature's remedies, there is no risk of repercussions of experimental backfiring.

The adrenal glands appear to have considerably more need for vitamin C and the B complex group, as well as vitamin A.

Reflexes to the adrenals will be the same as the kidneys, being found almost in the center of each foot just a bit up from the waistline of the foot. (See Chart 3.) If using the Reflex Massager be sure not to overmassage for the first week, since they cannot be massaged without massaging the reflex to the kidneys, which can be manipulated too much at first.

The pancreas is a larger gland lying in the back of the stomach and measuring some 6 to 8 inches in length. It produces pancreatic juice which it discharges through the pancreatic duct into the duodenum, the beginning of the intestine as it starts at the pyloric end of the stomach.

Pancreatic juice is essential to the conversion of consumed starch into maltose, a type of sugar; of fats into fatty acids and glycerol; of proteins into amino acids, these to be reassembled into the specific types of proteins or tissues as needed by the body for growth and repair.

This is the important gland that secretes insulin, which is widely recognized as necessary for the utilization of sugar into the production of energy.

The pancreas is an unusually sensitive organ and its slightest impairment will alter the chemistry of the body which may become subject to fluctuations of a particularly distressing character.

This is the gland that must function perfectly or the result is diabetes. It has been found that the heavy, fat-consuming nations and peoples of the world suffer the most from diabetes. It has also been found that synthetic corn sugar induces diabetes in test animals. The only specific need of the pancreas that is now known, other than an ordinary healthy diet, is the mineral zinc, which seems to be much less than normal in this gland when there is diabetes present.

To keep the pancreas in functioning, healthy condition, be sure to massage its reflex. It is in almost the same place as that of the kidneys and adrenals. It should get its proper share of stimulation when using the Reflex Massager. But if there is diabetes, beware of overmassaging this particular spot at first. Watch insulin intake, as it will stimulate the pancreas to produce insulin naturally and it is possible you will not need to take as much because of this.

One diabetic said that he had to cut down over half of his intake of insulin after the second treatment, and he had been taking it for over 20 years!

Gonads

As has been stated, the gonads are the sex glands: ovaries in the female, testes in the male. (See Chart 3.)

These glands produce the sex hormones. There is one gland besides the gonads which produces sex hormones, and that is the adrenal gland or cortex. Sparkling eyes, luminosity, self-reliance, and self-assurance are all signs that the gonads are functioning properly. Their hormones create inner warmth in the system, preventing tendencies for inflexibility. They are responsible for the ability to attract others and retain affection. They make our personalities radiant and magnetic.

There is a close relationship between the pituitary and the gonads. It has been found that a failure of the pituitary gland acts the same as castration or ovariotomy.

When such a failure occurs in the young, the result is dwarfism, a tendency to gross obesity, and arrested sexual development.

Case Histories of Arthritis Healed

Some of the endocrine glands produce cortisone and other needed substances, many of them probably yet unknown to science. We still don't know all there is to know about the needs of the body, but when it becomes ill, then we do know that someplace some gland is not supplying something that the body needs to maintain it in perfect working order.

But when we stimulate these glands back into their normal, healthy condition by massaging the reflexes to them, naturally they will start producing the life-giving substances which the body has been missing. As the glands return to normal functioning, so the body will return to normal health.

So start working on the closest thing to Nature for a natural and sure healing — your feet!

Study Chart 3 on the endocrine glands and massage the reflexes to all of them every other day for the first two weeks, and while you are massaging the reflexes to them, don't neglect the other reflexes that are there in the bottom of each foot. Remember, when one instrument is out of tune in the orchestra, it throws the rest of the instruments off and we have a song of discord. The body must be in harmony to give you the perfect health that everyone has the right to as long as he lives on this earth. Every truly healthy person should experience a feeling of exuberance and well-being all day through and be able to fall into a deep, painless sleep as soon as he gets into bed at night.

Is this the way you feel? If it isn't, then you are not enjoying the health that Nature intended you to have when you were born. All you have to do is TRY! Seek for health and it shall be given to you.

Take up your feet and start on the road to health Nature's way.

I presume that you have one of your feet up into position for massaging. Let us start with the big toe and give it a thorough going over, especially in the center where the reflex to the pituitary gland lies. Then work on each toe and under each one, pressing in with the rolling motion and massaging each place in this manner. When you find an extremely tender spot be sure to give it a good massage, and then later return to it and massage it again, as this indicates trouble in the body. Never forget that although this massage makes the feet feel like new ones, our main concern is the healing of the body.

After you have worked over each toe and around it, move on down to the thyroid reflex just under the bone of the big toe, and massage it well, pressing in deeply so as to reach the parathyroids' reflexes. These are very important little glands, little but mighty, and you may have to use the Reflex Massager or a like device to reach them, as you can see in Chart 3 they are deeper than the thyroid and thus harder to reach. After the thyroids, move the fingers on to the adrenal gland reflex in the center of the foot and massage it, and then on to the sex glands under the ankles. Now, go back and cover the whole foot, massaging all of the rest of the reflexes. Never leave a tender spot in the foot unmassaged. Keep in mind if there is tenderness in the foot there is trouble in the body; so massage it out, even if you are not sure what part of the body it goes to. There is trouble there and you can relieve it by massaging the reflex that is telling you of it by giving pain sensations when you press in on it.

Don't neglect any part of the foot. When you have massaged it thoroughly, put it down and pick up the other foot, giving it the same treatment that you have just given this one.

Let me tell you of two people who came to me suffering with arthritis. There are so many who have been helped by massaging the reflexes for arthritis that I could write a book telling you about them.

A man was brought to me by his wife. He was so crippled with arthritis that he could hardly walk. He had to lean on his wife for support and then was only barely able to hobble into my office. I helped him into the chair and removed his shoes and stockings. His poor feet were so curled and misshapen that it was hard to tell where any certain reflex would be located in them. His hands were in the same condition, with the fingers curling in misshapen knobs into the palms of the hands. His face was drawn with pain and his eyes had the hopeless look of one who has suffered excruciating agony with no promise of relief.

He had earned his livelihood as a carpenter and now was unable to work and support his family. His wife had had to get out and work and they had eventually gone on Welfare, which hurt his pride. The worry only added to his troubles, because stress of any kind seems to add fuel to the fire, as they say, for any arthritis sufferer.

The doctors gave him no hope of relief from this terrible malady and they had spent all of their savings on doctors and medication for him. Luckily at that time the Welfare Agency recognized reflexology as a healing agent and paid for the treatments. Even though I would have given him the treatments anyway, many people are too proud to accept.

It was almost impossible to locate any certain reflex in his misshapen feet. They were very tender and I had to work very slowly and gently in under the twisted bones. As I worked, the feet seemed to become more relaxed. I feel that pain and worry cause a lot of undue tension on muscles and that helps pull the affected areas more out of shape than the arthritis sometimes. In his case I worked on the hands, too, giving just a few minutes to each foot and each hand.

After a few treatments his hands and feet started to improve. He said that the pain had been so relieved after the first treatment that he had slept the whole night through for the first time in months.

Of course, we know what wonders massaging the reflexes does in restoring the normal functions of the body, and in many cases the feeling of renewed hope has much to do with a rapid recovery. In releasing tensions and worry from the mind, the body has a chance to relax and start its way back to normal functioning as Nature intended it to.

It wasn't long after he first came to me that his hands and feet began to uncurl and straighten out like the petals of flowers. It was wonderful to watch him improve so rapidly. He was soon able to use his hammer once more and walk naturally on his feet again. You can imagine how elated and thankful he and his wife were. Nature works in wondrous ways if we just know how to give her a chance to rebuild our bodies. She knows what to do, did she not build our bodies in the first place?

A very wealthy lady who had arthritis so badly that she finally had to use a wheelchair came to see me. She was very lucky that she had a husband who devoted his time and money to her every need. He had taken his wife to any doctor who promised any relief at all for her. She had the most expensive medication money could buy, but when we become stricken with some bodily ailment we are helpless in Nature's hands and sometimes all the money in the world cannot buy what Nature gives freely.

This lady's knees and ankles were swollen beyond belief. She suffered excruciating agony 24 hours a day, and her devoted husband's face was drawn with pain and worry in his suffering for her. Sometimes we suffer more for a loved one than we do for our own physical pain.

One might have thought her case was hopeless upon seeing the inflamed, swollen joints of this lovely woman as she was wheeled into the office. But as long as a person has hope there is always a chance, and if they keep searching they will find a way, Nature's way, usually after all other methods have been tried and have failed.

Did she respond to the reflexology treatments? It was like watching a miracle unfold before your eyes at her rapid recovery after a few weeks of treatments. Today she is free of pain, and to see her walking down the street in her fancy dress shoes, one would never think that such a very short time ago she had been an invalid, racked with pain.

If reflexology can do this for others, it can do it for you. And don't get discouraged. Remember, you took a long time to get into the condition that you are in now, so how can you expect Nature to completely cure you in a few days or even weeks? Keep up your hope and don't get discouraged. The symptoms of arthritis have a bad habit of getting better for a while and raising people's hopes, then letting them down by flooding back with all of the old miseries. In the reflexology treatments, I notice that this surging back and forth of the disease is much less than with other types of treatments, and the improvements seem to be more steady. But if it doesn't happen to you, don't give up! Remember, a tree doesn't grow in a day, but patience will prevail.

CHAPTER 26

Reflex Tonics for Overcoming Fatigue

Chronic fatigue is the curse of our modern age. In this day of increased leisure and labor-saving gadgets, everyone crowds his allotted 24 hours with hectic activity, which results in both physical and mental weariness. Many doctors report that their patients complain of "being tired," even when the doctors are unable to find any medical reason for it. Through reflex massage, however, fatigue can be relieved quickly and easily at any time, anywhere, by everyone. Let us look at a few typical cases of average people in routine situations.

The Busy Housewife

Let's suppose that you have been rushed all day, cleaning and dusting and preparing a gourmet dinner for invited guests. As the hour approaches for their arrival, you suddenly feel "beat" and have no energy left for serving and entertaining, for being a beautiful and charming hostess. You think, "If there only were some kind of magic tonic to give me an instant pickup!" Well, you do have one, right there on the bottom of your little, pink feet.

The Pituitary

Sit down in the nearest chair, and kick off your shoes. Lift one foot up into position (either one will do). Now, give the center of

153

your big toe a quick massage, remembering to press deeply enough to touch the reflex to the pituitary gland. Then move on down to the thyroid reflex, which is just under the bone of the big toe. If you have remembered which chart, you will know just where to massage. If you haven't, refer to it for best results.

The Adrenals

Next, move your fingers back toward the center of the sole to find the reflexes to the adrenal glands. These are the quick-energy glands for the magic tonic you need right *now*. They boost vigor and promote your inner drive to action, the glands that give you untiring energy. Massage them about 30 seconds only — remember, you are looking for *a fast pickup* and not a general health treatment. You will feel an immediate recharging of your worn down body batteries.

Sex Glands

The gonads, or sex glands, are also important in depleting our energies, and as I stated in the chapter on glands, the adrenal glands also produce sex hormones. It is from these hormones that you get sparkling eyes and self-reliance, and they make for a radiant and magnetic personality. So, continue with the massage by moving your fingers to the ankle area, and massage the reflexes which lie just under the ankle bones on the top area of the foot. After about 15 seconds of massage, change to the other foot and massage it the same way: first, the pituitary in the large toe; then the thyroid; next, the adrenal; and finally the ankle for the sex glands.

Conditioning the Spleen

Now, there is one more important reflex to massage — that for the spleen. The spleen is the storage container of our life energy forces, and the producer of red blood cells. It is on the left side only, so take your foot into position and place your fingers just under the little toe. (This is the reflex to the heart.) Move just below this pad, and massage immediately under it to find the reflex to the spleen.

Massage this reflex for about 30 seconds, and while you are in this area, you may as well give the heart an extra boost, too, with 15 or 20 seconds of massage.

Final Brushups

Finally, go back and give the reflex to the pituitary on the center of the big toe an extra deep prod or two, as a final signal for it to get busy and help the other glands send you some quick energy.

Complete the treatment by rotating each foot vigorously a few times, using a rolling motion, first to the left and then to the right.

The whole procedure should have taken you less than five minutes, and believe me, you will find that you never spent a more rewarding five minutes, especially when your husband compliments you at the end of an enchanting evening and wonders how you did it all and still managed to look beautiful and full of youthful energy.

Consider the Family

Try to keep in mind that other members of the family may be suffering from fatigue without being aware of the reason for their irritability, accompanied by a feeling of futility and depression. There can be no doubt that a constant, nagging sense of fatigue can develop into man's greatest enemy to happy, joyful living. It has been known to wreck homes, to shorten life, and it certainly makes life far from enjoyable. It can lead to mental illness. Frequently, it means being more weary on rising than on going to bed and dragging a heavy, overtaxed body around day after day. How pointless it is to allow such a situation to continue when reflexology provides fast, cost-free relief!

Restoring the Bread Winner's Energies

Let's turn our focus on the man-of-the-family who may feel unwilling to admit that he is not quite the tower of strength he pretends to be. In his desperate need for sufficient strength to carry through day after day, he may be driven to pep pills or alcoholic drinks which not only provide relief for a very short duration but may also adversely affect his personality. His fatigue may spring from any number of causes. He may snatch a hasty meal which does not contain sufficient nourishment. He may be under constant mental or physical pressure. Long driving through heavy traffic to and from work adds to the drain of energy. When he arrives at home, he may collapse into a comfortable chair and fall asleep. It is a sign that somewhere the generators of the electric forces are not functioning at their full efficiency, that his cells are dying and the process of age is creeping in faster than it should.

Here is where the knowledgeable wife takes action to restore him to youthful vitality.

Remove his shoes and socks, and bathe his feet with a cool washcloth which has been saturated with a mild mixture of vinegar and water. Then proceed to give him a quick pickup reflex massage as outlined in the beginning of this chapter. Watch the change in him and his feelings toward you, as weariness makes room for a new surge of energy which floods his entire body as if by a miracle.

In addition to this fast pickup treatment, a complete reflex massage of both feet to recondition the body can be given just before retiring for the night, or at a time when it can be followed by sleep for an hour or longer.

There is no reason, of course, why the man of the house should not help his wife restore her own depleted energies after a hectic day at home with its many demands on her strength. It will result in maintaining a cheerful disposition, as by day's end her nerves may be frazzled.

Let me say in conclusion to wives and brides, that if you want your husband to come running home to you past all the temptations on the way for the rest of your life, the key to that secret is a reflexology pickup when he gets home from the day's work.

What to Do for Exhausting Shopping Trips

Shopping trips can be real energy robbers. Assume that you and a friend start out fresh and enthusiastic, for a day of shopping. You walk the streets, going from store to store, searching for just the right dress, or furniture, or whatever. After hours of tramping, there comes a time when you feel ready to collapse on the street, and your enthusiasm is all gone. You haven't found what you were looking for, after all. Your muscles are protesting, and your head is beginning to ache. What can you do for a quick pepper-upper? Take a reflexology tonic as indicated in this chapter.

Find a lounge in one of the stores, or go to your car if you prefer. Take your shoes off and massage those pep-restorer reflexes mentioned above.

A Case History of Overcoming Shopping Exhaustion

As proof of the effectiveness of this treatment, let me tell you about a personal experience. With a close friend, I drove about 100 miles to a large city to attend an evening concert. We left early in the morning so that we would have a leisurely day for shopping.

At about one o'clock, my friend began to complain about a headache. She grew more and more tired, and we had to look for a place where she could rest. I offered to massage her feet if we could find a place where she could sit down. She kept insisting that she would be fine after taking some pills. But before long she felt so weak and exhausted that we went into a lounge in one of the stores, where she collapsed into a chair. I removed her shoes and massaged the reflexes to the glands that produce quick energy, and also her big toe to relieve the headache.

While we were doing this, one of the clerks came in. She said, "That looks wonderful to me — I think I'll pull off my shoes and have you rub my feet, too." She seemed to sense instinctively that rubbing the feet is relaxing.

After rubbing my friend's feet, I let her rest quietly for about five minutes. Her headache vanished completely, and she was soon filled with renewed vigor. "It's like getting your second wind," she commented. We finished shopping, enjoyed a wonderful concert, and drove 100 miles home late in the evening, all without suffering from the "drag" that often spoils an otherwise pleasant excursion.

Quick Energy Pickup for Travel Exhaustion

You may be a traveling salesman, or just one of those unfortunate people who cannot take very much traveling without feeling drained of all energy after a few hours of driving or riding. Or, perhaps you are a senior citizen who would like to take one of those interesting bus excursions but do not feel that you have the energy to travel that far.

In whatever category you are, even if there is no one available who can give you a fast reflex massage, by studying the charts and applying the simple techniques of foot reflexology, you can help yourself to renewed energy and a feeling of well-being. And this can be done without resorting to drugs or other artificial pep-boosters which leave you in the same weary condition, if not worse, when their effects wear off.

Reflexology Tips When Traveling with the Family

The average vacationing family tries to cover too many miles in a hurry, with the result that the children get restless and tired. Traveling with a family means many hectic demands on mind and body, not only for the driver but for everyone who accompanies him. It is no wonder that too many people simply say, "It isn't worth it!" But if everyone in the family learns the way to give a fast pickup by massaging the reflexes of the feet, any vacation can be a pleasant experience!

When the children become irritable and restless, have them give each other a foot massage which will quiet them down. In the evening, take turns massaging each other's feet, and you will enjoy a good night's rest and wake ready for another memorable day.

But let me give you a word of caution: *don't forget that this treatment is very relaxing even if given for only a few seconds.* This is fine for the children for they will fall asleep, or at least be less quarrelsome. But if the treatment lasts more than five minutes, be sure that you can lie down and sleep for an hour or so before trying to drive again.

Although a quick pepper-upper treatment can be given any time weariness begins to set in, the best time for a good overall treatment is just before going to bed. You will be so relaxed that you will sleep like a baby, as the saying goes. And you will also wake up in the morning with all the bounce and energy of youth and be able to look forward to all those miles ahead with anticipation and eagerness.

Reflexology for Campers

A pickup tonic through foot reflexology is exactly what every amateur outdoor sportsman is looking for after a hard day's tramping the hills trying to locate that invisible deer, that covey of quail, or flush pheasants out of cover; or the fisherman who has put in many hours from before daylight climbing over miles of rocks trying to hook that granddaddy trout just beyond the next bend; or the duck hunter who comes in cold, wet, and exhausted after hours of sitting in the rain, cramped in a blind on the marshy shore of a lake.

Your first move in getting back to camp is to get out of your wet clothes immediately. If a meal is ready for you, sit down and eat. If not, and you are too tired to fix something, turn to the feet for a fast camper's pickup tonic!

It is better to have someone else give you a treatment, one who understands the technique of reflex massage. But if necessary, then give yourself a treatment.

Take off your shoes and socks, and start massaging the feet as described. If you are very cold and your feet are wet, just rub them briskly for a few minutes before starting to massage the reflexes. You will be surprised to see how quickly this warms you all over, and after digging and prodding and massaging the reflexes in both feet, you will feel a warm glow spreading over your entire body.

If you do not intend to go to bed right away, however, do not massage the entire foot as you will become very sleepy. For just a quick energy pickup, massage the big toe and under it, then the center section of the bottom of both feet (for the adrenal glands), under the ankle bones (for the gonads), and on the left foot under the little toe pad for the spleen and the heart — which, incidentally, is good to massage whenever you are out exerting yourself in ways your body is not accustomed to, in order to give it an extra boost of stimulation.

Heart Attacks While Out in the Field

The opening day of hunting and fishing or any other sporting season is sure to bring countless reports of sudden heart attacks suffered by sportsmen of all ages. Long periods of inactivity have left the heart unprepared for the sudden surge of adrenalin which is rushed to this blood-pumping organ at the first sign of excitement. Remember that the heart is really a large muscle, and that an easy life keeps it pumping slowly. Thus it becomes soft from lack of exercise, just like any other muscle which has become weakened under routine demands. When the adrenal gland is stimulated by excitement, the heart speeds up its rhythm and pumps at a much faster rate. Sometimes it cannot take such a sudden change of pace without causing great discomfort or even a heart attack.

If a heart attack should occur when the victim is miles away from a doctor, first massage the reflex under the little toe of the left foot, and then continue to massage all over this toe including the area on top of it. Then move to the reflex of the pituitary in the center of the big toe for a few seconds of massage, and return to the little toe area.

It is, in fact, a good idea to give yourself a reflex massage any time that you feel odd in any way while out hiking. Just sit down, take off your shoes, and rub the area around your little toe and under it for a few minutes. Dig in deeply, even if you have to use a stick. Or, if there is a rocky area nearby, walk over it in your bare feet. Of course, it will hurt! But that is better than having a disabling illness strike you, isn't it? It may forestall an impending heart attack, and in any event, it will recharge your vitality and give you strength either to get to a doctor or to go on with the hike if you are merely fatigued.

Reflexology for Leg Cramps

Leg cramps in muscles unused to sudden demands are a common complaint of outdoorsmen and others. Familiarity with foot reflexology is the answer to get fast relief.

A few years ago a friend and I took our places near a certain path early one morning, to wait for a large buck which came down the mountain every day just about dawn. We sat motionlessly, watching the trail. Just when it was time for the deer to show, my friend whispered, "I have a terrible cramp in my leg. I'm sorry, but I've just got to move." Both of us realized that to make a move at that crucial moment would give our presence away. I reached over quietly and massaged the cords in back of his knee for a few minutes. This relaxed the cramped muscles in his leg, and he was able to sit patiently until the unsuspecting deer appeared in sight. Without a knowledge of foot reflexology, we would have missed getting the biggest trophy of the hunting trip.

Hot Weather Fatigue

Does hot weather leave you depleted of energy? Foot reflexology is the answer. If you are not one of those fortunate people who can boast that they "thrive" on hot weather, chances are you suffer from the fagged feeling known as "heat exhaustion."

When a hot day drains you of energy, just find a nice, shady nook, bare your feet if they are not already bare, and give them a massage that will stimulate the glands that recharge the entire body, as stated in this book.

Massage the reflex to the pituitary gland in the center of the big toe to stimulate it into action so that it can start sending energy to the thyroid, adrenals, spleen, and gonads. Once you get them into action, they will stimulate the rest of the body.

In this chapter, you have been given the "recipe" for a fast pickup tonic to use whenever you feel low in vitality. Apply the same method of massage to the same glands for hot weather fatigue, and you will feel refreshed and invigorated as if by magic.

CHAPTER 27

How to Have More "Go Power" with Reflexology

I have told you so much about how to relax, and how to overcome various illnesses, now I would like to tell you how to use reflexology as your "go power," how to recharge your vitality and give you a pickup that will last all day.

How to Get Started for the Day

One of my patients told me that she had a hard time getting up in the mornings. "It just seems that I couldn't get awake, or make my body respond without a great effort," she said. "Then I would wander around in a daze for an hour or more before I could get in gear and move and think normally. One morning I had a lot of work ahead of me. As I opened my eyes I thought of all the work I had to get done that day and I wished that I could feel full of pep and vitality and be able to jump out of bed and pitch into it, instead of dragging around for an hour drinking coffee for a stimulant.

"As I lay there I thought of reflexology. If it worked to relax you when you were tired, why couldn't it pep you up when you needed a stimulant in the morning?" She went on to tell me that she curled around in bed and started to massage her feet as I had shown her. "I decided if the pituitary reflex relaxed, then it should also be able to give me some 'go power,' so I gave both big toes a good working over. Then I worked my thumb on down under the big toe bone where you had shown me the reflex to the thyroid was located and gave that a couple of pushes. If anyone ever needed a push button to start their motor going with a zing, I needed it this particular morning, so I covered my feet quickly with the rolling push-and-pull motion that you had taught me. I don't think the whole procedure took me over two minutes, but by the time I was finished, I felt wide awake. I got out of bed and was so full of energy I started in on my work before I realized that I had not had my coffee yet. No more lying in bed dreading to get up for me," she said. "I felt wonderful the whole rest of the day."

The massaging of these reflexes in the bottom of your feet is like opening up a new power within you. Nearly everyone today knows that we are filled with a great power likened to T.N.T. — yes, even the atomic bomb, which is merely atoms exploding for the will of man.

Our bodies are as subject to the rhythmic laws of Nature and the universe as the planet is in its revolution around the sun.

Everything is in a state of vibration. There is nothing in absolute rest; from the greatest sun to the tiniest atom, there is motion and vibration, just as the atoms of the human body are in constant vibration and change. Do you know that if one single atom were deprived of vibration it is said that it would wreck the universe? Matter is being constantly played upon by energy and countless forms result, and yet even the forms are not permanent; they begin to change the moment they are created and from them are born new forms, which in turn change and give rise to newer forms, and so on.

The atoms in the human body are in constant vibration. Changes are occurring unceasingly. There is almost a complete change in the matter composing the body within a few months. There will scarcely be a single atom now composing your body, found a few months from now. Nothing is permanent in the world of forms; they are but appearances and they come and they go — constant vibration — constant change.

Reflexology, the Natural Primer

So in reflexology we have the natural method of sending these powerful vibrations to any spot in our body, thus recharging the atoms with a shot of T.N.T. through the reflexes. We might say we are transferring the power in any atom in our bodies to places where we need a burst of energy for a quick pickup or to stimulate the atoms in a certain sluggish area to a new surge of circulation, life, and energy. If the matter of our bodies is in constant change at a certain rate of vibration, then you can easily see how simple it is for Nature to heal any and all dissensions in the body if given a chance to vibrate in rhythm. In all vibration there is found to be a certain rhythm. Rhythm pervades the universe.

So we turn to reflexology and massage the reflexes in the bottoms of the feet to get the body back into its natural rhythm with the universe.

Our bodies are as subject to rhythmic laws as is the planet in its revolution around the sun.

If a high note is sounded repeatedly and in rhythm, it will start into motion vibrations that can bring down a building. Even soldiers marching in rhythm across a bridge will set up vibrations that could bring the bridge down. These manifestations of the effect rhythmic motion has on matter will give you an idea of how important rhythm and harmony is to the health of our bodies. If we are out of rhythm, then there can be no harmony. Our bodies are made to harmonize with the universal vibratory rhythm of this planet on which we live, and you can readily see how out of balance your whole body can become if you allow it to be filled with things of disharmonious vibrations.

This is why so many people seemingly have every gland and organ in their body malfunctioning in one way or another. How can a body run smoothly and in perfect health if the instruments are out of tune, such as the glands and the organs? Any one of them can start a chain reaction of disharmony and illness. So many people come to me with the same story, "I don't know what is the matter with me. I am just sick all over. The doctors don't know either; they say it is my mind. But I can't eat; if I do, it makes me sick. I am losing weight and I have no energy to go as I used to."

Why the Whole Body Must Be Reflexed

These people cannot be helped by just treating one part of the body. All of the body has become out of tune and the vibrations of its atoms are not changing in a perfect pattern of health, because somewhere some gland has been allowed to get out of harmony. To have perfect health throughout the body, we will have to get our vibrations back into rhythm and our glands and organs back into tune with each other so that they can send harmonious vibrations into every atom that is busy trying to build the body back to the full strength of every cell.

This is why reflexology brings about such seeming miracles. Actually it is a very simple and natural process of tuning the instruments of the body; just press the reflexes in the bottoms of the feet to break up the congestion that has accumulated there, thus slowing down the circulation of the life forces to certain glands and organs. All of the cells in the body will be energized by the radiations of vital force emitted from these glands when the reflexes are used to awaken them back to their natural functions.

I am telling you these natural workings of Nature's laws so that you will realize the simplicity and yet the power of using reflexology to regain your health, and to keep your body in perfect harmony and health for as long as you live.

By massaging the reflex to the pituitary you are tuning the main gland, as you would tune the leading violin in a symphony orchestra. This is the way our bodies harmonize with the symphony of the universe when they are in perfect tune. But have you ever heard an orchestra tuning their instruments? Or can you imagine how an orchestra would sound if just one instrument were out of tune? Can you see how impossible it is for us to have good health and energy if some part of our body has gotten out of tune?

Reflexology is the only method I know of that works on the whole body at the same time, leaving no instrument or gland untouched, as the feet are completely covered by massage. There is no part left out unless you miss it as you massage the whole of the left foot and the whole of the right foot.

The pituitary gland, which has its reflex in the center of the big toe, is the pep gland. It also has a direct bearing on the sex glands which are responsible for our personalities and our drive, our get-up-and-go, our vitality and energy.

How Reflexology Revitalizes All of You

You will find that the men or women who are very successful will be the ones with a strong sex drive; and the endocrine glands have to be in good health for them to have this sex drive. If you are not mentally alert and don't want to work for success, then you probably lack a strong sex drive and will be content to sit and let the world go by, unless you stimulate the endocrine glands to normal action. And the most natural and most simple way to do this is by massaging the reflexes to all of these glands.

We have discussed the pituitary gland and its reflexes in the big toe. The next gland is also in the head and is massaged in the big toe also, only instead of in the center, we move the finger over to the side toward the second toe to find the reflex to the pineal gland. If the reflex to the pituitary is tender, then this will also probably be quite sensitive when pressed on. Then we go to the reflexes to the thyroid gland just under the bone of the big toe, and the parathyroids in the same location as the thyroid. However, the parathyroids are deeper and more pressure must be put into the massaging of them if they need special attention, otherwise they will receive enough stimulation as you massage the thyroid reflexes.

The thymus is important, too, and will have a reflex in the center of each foot almost up at the root of the toes.

Then we go to the adrenals, the reflexes being in the center of each foot. And remember, they, like the sex glands, give you go power, drive to act, untiring activity.

Then we have the pancreas gland which is larger than the other endocrine glands which lies behind the lower part of the stomach. This is the gland that produces insulin, among other things. Anyone suffering from diabetes is familiar with the feeling of weakness suffered when this gland is not working properly and fails to supply a sufficient amount of insulin. So we would massage the reflexes to this all-important gland in the center of each foot above the reflex to the adrenal glands. Since it is in the same position as the stomach, it will get the benefit of the massage when you massage the stomach; and in doing this particular reflex massage you also help digestion in two ways, as the pancreas is also a producer of pancreatic juice containing enzymes which are important in digestion.

Then we go to the gonads (sex glands) and massage the reflexes to them, as you will remember, in the area of the ankles.

It is well to massage all around the ankles on the inside and outside of both feet, and up the back of the leg just above the heel on both sides of the cord extending up the back of the leg, as this whole area has reflexes to the reproductive glands.

In massaging the whole foot, all of the cells will be stimulated as the circulation is released to allow the natural life force to bring renewed vigor to every part of the body. In this way the vibrations of the life force will bring harmony and health back to every part of the body.

The little gland called the spleen is not only a builder of red blood cells to keep you full of health and pep, but it is also a storehouse of the life force that we receive from the surrounding air. Medical centers seem to have little understanding of this life force as yet, which is called "prana" by the yogis. But it is truly an electrical life force and without it nothing could live.

So keep your spleen healthy by massaging the reflex to it which is located under the reflex to the heart, on your left foot. See Chart 2 for exact location to massage. When one uses a Reflex Massager, the whole foot is more easily and thoroughly covered, thus insuring that all the reflexes have been amply massaged.

When this life force is distributed over the entire body through the etheric networks, it radiates on the surface of the body as an aura of health. If you want your aura to be colored with perfect health and energy and your body to vibrate in tune with the symphony of the universe, keep it in perfect condition by massaging the reflexes in the bottoms of your feet as indicated in this book.

CHAPTER 28

How Mental Health Can Be Improved with Reflexology

As we have seen in this book, the body is not merely a machine which gets out of order here and there, but a delicately balanced system which must function smoothly and efficiently, and the degree of its efficiency seems to have a direct connection with one's mental health. Conversely, a state of worry, tension, anxiety, etc., can affect various organs and glands and bring on distressing physical ailments. So dependent and inseparable are the two aspects of man, mental and physical, that many cases of nervousness, indigestion, premature senility, irritability, depression, and even some cases of mental retardation, have their origin in a malfunctioning body.

Reflex massage is Nature's own method of restoring the body to full efficiency, which in turn has a beneficial effect on the personality as tensions give way to peace of mind.

The Rule of Relaxation for Mental Health

The first rule toward regaining peace of mind is relaxation, but one cannot relax when the body is shouting protests, and how can a person radiate love and harmony if the mind is in a turmoil? The most common remedy for physical or mental distress is to put something in the mouth instead of attacking the source, and relief always seems to be just around the corner in the next drugstore.

Now, we all know that there is no miracle pill that can really relieve the body of strain or the mind of stress except temporarily. Our environment has become so complicated that many people live in a state of fear and are willing to try almost anything for escape. Some turn to sedatives or alcohol, some find refuge in cigarettes, watching fights, gambling — whatever diverts the attention momentarily. Some take up causes, or sex, or war, or even religion. A few are driven to that final resort, suicide. Still, man's problem is not solved, and will remain unresolved until he turns within himself to find the answers. To be able to relax for quiet meditation, he must be relaxed not only in mind but in body as well.

In this push-button age, we have overlooked Nature's own push buttons, right in the bottom of the feet. All you have to do is push them or walk on them on a rough surface. What could be simpler and more rewarding than this simple but powerful push-button method which takes care of the body and the mind at the same time?

Reflex Massage for Mental Benefits

Those who turn to reflex massage, Nature's own marvelous invention, will come closest to discovering the freedom for which they are searching. With renewed joy and youthful vigor, the disposition improves, efficiency increases, tasks are approached with eagerness and not apprehension, and the whole personality radiates love and optimism.

The vibrations that you send up to the pituitary gland with reflexology are filled with a power that will blend the whole system into harmony — and all you have to do is press the reflex button in the center of your big toe to start the vibrations of health swinging into action. It is no wonder that this pituitary gland is called the "king gland"!

Then, as you proceed to massage the other reflexes, you will feel an immediate response as the process of eliminating poisons from your system commences. Remember that you are awakening sluggish glands and freeing them from the congestions that are affecting your very life. For this reason, you must remember not to be overeager for faster results by overdoing the massage at first. Start the treatment gently for a few seconds, then wait two or three days before the next one to give the body time to readjust itself. Just as a champion runner must train his muscles gradually, the body is in no condition to assume full efficiency without time.

How to Improve Your Disposition

The monotony and grind of household chores, the daily pressure of schedules, shopping, etc., are a severe strain on the average homemaker. The vitality wanes, there are symptoms of mental fatigue, and she becomes cross, irritable, and unpleasant. Her temper flares at the children and her hapless husband, and she often goes from aspirin to sleeping pills for relief from nervous headaches and insomnia. Marriage seems to have become a trap from which there is no escape.

Reflexology Break vs. Coffee Break

There is no need for allowing such a mental condition to develop. Instead of a "coffee break" or a dose of sedatives, take a reflexology break and see how quickly you feel a recharge of vitality rushing through you. The reflex buttons in the bottoms of your feet are there as a gift from Nature to give you an energy boost any time you need it. All you have to do is sit down for five minutes and massage them for a fast pickup, and you will receive as an extra bonus a wonderful feeling of well-being. You will no longer feel trapped but will see life through rose-colored glasses and be restored to health and vigor, with a calm, happy, understanding disposition. The woman of the house needs to remain strong in body as well as good-natured, cool, and beautiful.

The Disposition of the Male

And all this goes for men as well. When a man comes home cranky and irritable, it is hard for the children and his wife to greet him warmly.

He comes in, banging the door in a rage about some small thing that happened at the office, or perhaps the paper was torn by the pup. No wonder the children stand in awe of him, or watch carefully to see what mood he is in, or just make themselves scarce when he comes home. Does this sound like you? This is not the real you, and it is not the way you want your home life to be but somehow you have gotten into a rut. The daily "rat-race" of earning a living, trying to keep up with the times which means buy-buy-buy, bigger bills, and higher taxes, give you reason to worry, right? But why ruin your life worrying? Everything works out, given time.

Do you realize that if every gland and organ in your body were in complete harmony with the universe and functioning properly, you would not let even the big things get you down, let alone life's minor irritations?

Do you come home with a smile on your face and a song in your heart? Do you radiate a happy attitude and fill the house with the warmth of your personality?

No one can have a sunny disposition if he is feeling under par. Tension from fear and worry can and does throw the body out of chemical balance. It tends to weaken the whole human organism, *especially the adrenal glands,* and if the supply of adrenal hormones runs dry, it can lead to various crippling diseases. Even though there is no sudden attack of illness of any kind, the body has actually been under a period of deterioration possibly for many years. A relaxed mind leads to relaxed nerves, and relaxed nerves make for a healthy body and a pleasant disposition.

"But how can I get rid of my worries and tensions?" You ask. *It is so simple, once you know the secrets of reflexology.* You can press a few buttons while relaxing in front of the T.V. and regain all the pep and vigor of youth, in a few minutes of massage once or twice a week. Why not use it to catapult yourself into a new way of life and become the true person you were meant to be, and that your family certainly wants you to be? Instead of a coffee break or a beer break, try a reflexology break first and enjoy life to its very fullest for the rest of your life. This book can show you the way to do it.

Extreme Mental Cases Helped

Through my years of treating people with reflexology, I came across many cases of mental stress — some of them minor and some so serious as to require commitment to an asylum. A colleague told me of cases which she had treated who were patients, some so agitated that they had become dangerous. With reflex massage, she had been able to restore some of them to the point where they could return home.

I remember one case of mine whose family did not want to have committed. His wife asked me to come to the house to see if reflexology could be of any help.

"We don't really think that just rubbing the feet will do much good, but we are willing to try anything," she commented.

When I arrived, Mrs. D. met me at the door, her eyes filled with fear and exhaustion. Mr. D. was still a young man, and had been teaching school. He had become increasingly nervous and irritable the past few months, and the school was finally forced to ask him to take a leave of absence. Now he was having spells of violence and didn't seem to know what he was doing. The doctor prescribed sedatives, but he refused to take them. She had become so afraid of him that she had sent the children to stay with her mother.

"I'm afraid to let you go in," said Mrs. D. as she led me to the bedroom.

"Now, you leave me alone with him, and don't worry," I said. "I will be able to handle him, and I'll have him like a lamb in no time!" I could see a faint glimmer of hope light up in her eyes as I went into the room and closed the door.

The room was a mess, and so was Mr. D. He needed a haircut and a shave. His bedding was scattered on the floor, and he had torn his night clothes to shreds. He looked as if he had reverted to an animal. His eyes were wild as if he were trapped and ready to spring at me any moment.

I felt a deep pity for this poor, mentally disturbed man, but no fear as I talked gently to him, telling him that I had come to rub his feet and relieve his tensions. I kept repeating that rubbing his feet would make him feel relaxed and help him to sleep. He watched me, wild eyed, as I approached slowly to the bed where he crouched ready to bolt and run. He didn't move, however, as I sat on the edge of the bed, carefully took one of his feet in my hands, and began rubbing it very gently. He began to relax a little.

As soon as I felt that he was ready to trust me, I explained what I was going to do to his feet, and that it might hurt a little but that this was necessary to help him get well. He seemed to be listening intently, although his eyes still looked wild and untrusting.

Ever so lightly, I pressed on the reflex to the pituitary in the center of the big toe. As expected, it was very tender. He flinched but did not pull his foot away. I found the thyroid reflex very sensitive to pressure, as well as the adrenal and gonad reflexes. Also the reflex to the thymus was painful to the touch. I did not know exactly what this had to do with his condition, but there was definitely some connection there.

As I went over both feet gently, I found the reflexes on one foot more sensitive than the ones on the other. This seems to be general in cases of mental disorders.

I was unable to see if I had helped Mr. D. very much, but when I had completed a very short treatment, I suggested that he go to sleep now, and that I could come back to massage his feet again in two days. His eyes watched me warily but he did not offer to move from his position.

I told Mrs. D. that I thought he would sleep if left alone, and because she looked so harassed I talked her into letting me give her a quick reflex massage before I left.

Mrs. D. telephoned me the next day to say that she had lain down on the couch and gone to sleep, after I left, and when she woke up and looked in on her husband, he was sleeping soundly.

When I went back in two days as I had promised, I found Mr. D. sitting on the edge of the bed with a sheet pulled over him. I could see a glimmer of recognition in his eyes as he stretched out his foot to me. I pulled up a chair, and he quickly put both feet in my lap. He had remembered, and at least subconsciously knew that he had been helped, and that this was Nature's way of releasing his built-up tensions and distraught emotions.

I massaged the reflexes a little more severely this time since he didn't seem to mind. As I left, I told him I would return in two days.

To my surprise, on my third visit, I found both Mr. D. and Mrs. D. in the front room. Mr. D. was dressed and shaved.

"He still won't talk to me, or eat with me, but he keeps looking for someone. I'm sure it is you. I'm so thankful to you — I know you have saved his life," said Mrs. D.

"No, don't thank me," I said. "I only gave Nature a boost by massaging the reflexes as they were meant to be massaged in the first place. You could have done as much if you had understood about the reflexes and the technique of massaging them."

I suggested that we wait three days for the next treatment, and that we should see much improvement by then.

It was most gratifying to watch Mr. D.'s improvement after that, and he returned to teaching within six weeks.

I taught both Mr. and Mrs. D. how to keep the pituitary gland active and in good health by massaging the center of the big toe on each foot. I warned them that if at any time it showed the least tenderness, it must be massaged every other day or two until all tenderness had left.

There are, of course, those whom we cannot treat with such satisfying results, but still, reflexology can help to some extent and bring some semblance of relief.

A Case of Cerebral Palsy Helped

A boy was brought to my office so completely helpless that his mother had to carry him in from the car. He was 14 years of age, and had suffered from cerebral palsy from the time he was a baby. His body was terribly twisted, and he had no control over his arms, legs, or head. He had great difficulty in his speech but was able to say a few words with great effort.

When we put him in the chair the first time, he was very nervous and frightened, and asked if I were going to use an instrument. The boy had been to so many doctors and had been given so many shots and tests that he was frightened of everyone to whom his mother took him for treatment. She explained that there was just a chair for him to sit in, and one for me to sit on, and that there were no machines of any kind, but as she was not familiar with reflexology, she was unable to tell him what I was going to do.

When I lifted his feet into position for massage, I was shocked to see how twisted the poor things were. He seemed very frightened when I started to remove his shoes. I took time to explain that I was going to rub his feet, and that some of the places would hurt but all he had to do was tell me and I would be very gentle. I didn't know until later that the boy was also blind.

Of course, both his mother and I knew that reflexology would not cure him, but we also did not know how much help it could bring him. Since these children are very nervous, we hoped that it would at least be of some help. As soon as he understood that I would merely massage his feet, he relaxed and seemed to enjoy it.

His feet were so curled and misshapen that it was very difficult to work on them. In addition, they were in constant motion. There were no definite reflexes that I could work on except the toes and heel. However, I went over his feet the best I could, experimenting with the press-and-roll motion. In a case like this, we never know which reflex we might stimulate to give Nature's boost, thus starting a chemical reaction of the whole system that could restore health to parts of the body that were not recognized as being the seat of the ailment.

In treating with reflexology, I have learned to expect surprises of all kinds. In this case, the hands needed massage also, as they were so deformed and crippled that he was unable to hold anything, let alone be handled enough to stimulate the reflexes therein.

In this particular case, we felt that we may have improved his hearing, and to some extent his mental capacities. The treatments did help his nerves to a great extent, and also his disposition. My daughter, age 14, would come in after school and he showed an increasing interest in her and her chatter, and developed into one of the happiest-natured children I ever knew. Occasionally, I took other children to visit him.

How wonderful it would be if all those who are living restricted lives could be aided by reflexology toward a happier existence!

Overcoming Mental Depression

Although it is possible to obtain relief from physical discomforts through the techniques of reflexology, body tensions can result from poor thinking habits, and everyone should assume a cheerful, optimistic attitude toward life's problems and develop spiritual strengths by taking positive steps to learn as much as possible about God's great love for all His people. Every library and bookstore has many books on methods of acquiring such blessings as success, wealth, and happiness, as man's divine right. Man is not made to live in fear and want, in poor health, or a state of hopelessness. Reflexology can do much to change our desperate preoccupation with mental and physical discomforts without resorting to drugs or other escape routes.

We need only to observe words in common use to realize that body illnesses produce changes in personality. For instance, an irritable person is said to be "choleric." Through reflex massage, not only one's health but his personality can be changed for the better quickly and easily.

A Case of Depression Healed

One day a man came to the office, complaining that he felt very depressed, couldn't find any interest in life any more, and sometimes felt like "ending it all" as he was a "burden" to his family and friends.

As a matter of fact, he was not a burden to his family, and had many fine friends. He worked hard and supplied his family with luxuries, was apparently in good health, and had no special worries. The man had everything in the world to be thankful for, and here he was, talking of ending his life!

After talking with him for awhile, I asked him to sit in the chair and remove his shoes and socks. The first reflex I look for is the one to the pituitary gland in the center of the big toe. It was very tender, and he nearly jumped out of the chair. "What did you do — stick a needle in my toe?" he asked.

I explained that I had merely used the edge of my thumb to press into his toe, and that the "needle" he thought he felt was already inside the toe. I showed him how to do it for himself, and he was amazed at the painful result. I told him this was probably the cause of his unhappiness, the little culprit that was the source of his mental depression and loss of interest in life. I mentioned further that the pituitary was the "king gland" in his body and acted as a kind of harmonizer of the whole system, and that bullying, lying, vagrancy, and moroseness in children had been traced to a faulty pituitary gland through a course of experiments made by Dr. Rowe.

Also, I explained that the reflex to the pineal gland which was located in his big toe was another clue, as it is an organizer of harmony in the other endocrine glands, and that the improper functioning of these glands could be normalized by massaging the reflexes located in the bottom of the feet. He was very interested in my method of massage and asked me to proceed, no matter how painful it might be.

As I went over each reflex, I found the areas of the endocrine glands to be the most sensitive, but none was as tender as the one in the big toe. I kept returning to give it a few seconds of massage, and as I had learned to expect with anyone in his mental state, the reflex was more tender in one foot than in the other.

My patient became very relaxed, and on leaving, he said, "You know, I think the world looks better to me already! How soon can I come back?"

This man needed only six treatments in all, to restore his will to live and acquire a renewed zest for life.

He was so grateful for his new lease on life that he asked me to give him lessons on reflexology techniques. Now he devotes a lot of his own time massaging the reflexes of all who ask him for help with health problems.

And that is why I have written this book — so that you, too, can give yourself, or anyone else, a natural secret to health which will increase the circulation to glandular areas and promote health and efficiency of the glands and organs, resulting in a healthier, happier you.

Index